RUNNING

IS A

KIND OF

DREAMING

RUNNING
IS A
KIND OF
DREAMING

A Memoir

J. M. Thompson, PhD

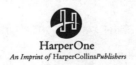

HarperOne
An Imprint of HarperCollinsPublishers

Grateful acknowledgment is made to the following for permission to reprint previously published material:

Page 37: Bobby Gosh, "Welcome to Our World Of Toys," copyright © 1986. Reprinted courtesy of Bygosh Music Corporation.

Page 69: Kurt Carr, "I Almost Let Go," copyright © 2008. Reprinted courtesy of Kcartunes (BMI) Lilly Mack Publishing (BMI) (administered at CapitolCMGPublishing).

Page 180: **Ac-cent-tchu-ate The Positive**
Lyric by Johnny Mercer
Music by Harold Arlen
© 1944 (Renewed) HARWIN MUSIC CO.
All Rights Reserved
Reprinted by Permission of Hal Leonard LLC

Page 251: Kyle David Matthews, "We Fall Down," copyright © 1997. Universal Music—Brentwood Benson Publishing (administered at CapitolCMGPublishing.com).

HarperCollins books may be purchased for educational, business, or sales promotional use. For information, please email the Special Markets Department at SPsales@harpercollins.com.

FIRST EDITION

Designed by Bonni Leon-Berman

Library of Congress Cataloging-in-Publication Data has been applied for.

ISBN 978-0-06-294707-9

21 22 23 24 25 LSC 10 9 8 7 6 5 4 3 2 1

For Shawn

See that all things are full of light. See the Earth, settled in the midst of the All, the great nurse who nourishes all terrestrial creatures. All is full of soul, and all beings are in movement.

—*Corpus Hermeticum XI: The Mind to Hermes*[1]

CONTENTS

Contents

AUTHOR'S NOTE

This is a work of nonfiction. In the course of writing these pages, I considered every salient trace of my past. In addition to my own memory, and the relevant scientific and philosophical literature, I reviewed multiple further sources, including letters, diaries, emails, photographs, videos, my medical records, and interviews with family members about their recollection of events at which they were also present. I have left nothing important out. I have not compressed multiple events into single scenes, created composite characters, or invented anything. I have represented dialogue to the best of my knowledge with fidelity. The following names are pseudonyms: Miriam, Chris, Don, Emily, Sebastian, Ned, Clara, Joseph, Dr. Jensen, Thelma, Dr. Browning, Dr. Hewitt, Mr. Butler, Roland, Mr. Martin, Sam, Mr. Keene, Sandra, Tara, Naomi, Mike, Andrew, Martha, Jim, and Dr. Carson. I have altered the names of some locations to protect the privacy of the individuals concerned.

—JMT

I

The Sun

Why

The trail leads into the quiet of the trees, the ancient ones, the womb of dirt and unseen birds, where no one knows my name: *Welcome, injured pilgrim.* Sugar pine, nuthatch, sierra juniper, the huff-puff of respiration, all the sad, mad, raging voices from the bad old days—everything transforms into the step before me and the instant I am in. Perhaps I have always been here, in this zone between the inner world and the outer one, where Earth in motion merges with mind and feeling and with all the times in memory and all the voids forgotten yet somehow sensed and known. The rhythm of my body, held within the blanket of the tree canopy, matches the music of the sparrow and the babble of the creek as all the mourning and madness turns into sweat and sunlight, and Earth moves under me and around me and within me. Hail, hawk and hummingbird. The leaves are whispering, *Hush now, little one, hush.* Hello, lupine, chickadee, thistle, blackbird, marten, nuthatch. Good morning, buttercup, yarrow, squirrel, robin, woodpecker. In the beginning there were no words, only sound and light and feeling, a rhythm of nothingness and being, and I feel it once more now in the sound of the wind, and in the pulse of sensing, again and again, the solid sentient core of an upright animal, accustomed to forest time. There is a path ahead of me. Nothing is ever altogether lost. There is a ground beneath us that never goes away.

IT'S AROUND ELEVEN IN the morning on a sunny Friday in the fall. I've climbed above the tree line and reached the high country. I'm about 5 miles into the Tahoe 200, a 205-mile ultramarathon on the rugged mountain trail around the largest alpine lake in North America. I've been running ultramarathons for a decade, but never this far. Right now I'm running on a ridge about two thousand feet above the lake. The lake looks back at me with its sparkling turquoise eye. The land below stretches to a faraway horizon as my body floats down the trail. I can feel the sunshine warm my face and hear the trees dancing in the wind with a sound like the cosmos breathing life into the world. The land and sky are shining as if someone has turned up all the colors of the world. The flowers look as bright and cheery as a bunch of little munchkins. Seeing Earth at this scale does something to the eye. Your focus shifts from the world up close to a bigger picture. Climb a little closer to our friendly neighborhood star and the mind shifts out of clock time into a timeless way of being.

I drove to Lake Tahoe with my wife, Miriam, and our son and daughter from our home in San Francisco around lunchtime yesterday. I love coming back to Tahoe. When I see the lake, I remember all the other times I've been here. The memories spiral on top of one another. Everywhere I look, *now* has *then* folded up inside it. Yesterday afternoon, gazing across the vast, still, blue surface of the water at the snow-flecked mountains on the other side, for a second I glimpsed the lake in my mind's eye, the way I saw it for the first time, eighteen years before. As I kept staring at the water, my mind spun back and forth between two bodies of water, one in the present and the other in memory, like two circles overlapping and then merging into one. "You're running around all of *that*?" my daughter said, looking at the lake and the distant mountains surrounding it. "Yes," I said. "Why?" she said.

Two hundred miles: it is the kind of distance you see on a freeway sign. Am I out of my mind? Not anymore. Ultrarunning can sound like insanity to people who don't do it. But ultrarunners understand its mad logic: running for days and nights nonstop brings you right up to the edge of breakdown but also to the opportunity for breakthrough. It's chaos, in a container: a kind of organized insanity that can help keep you sane. Still, I understand the optics of lunacy. I once heard a story about a group of runners in a café in a little mountain town. The runners were chatting about their plan to get up at four in the morning and run for thirty-six hours straight in the hills. A person at another table in the café overheard their conversation. "That sounds completely *unnecessary*," he said. And so it is. On the surface, an ultramarathon is neither necessary nor reasonable. And yet men and women in the tens of thousands appear compelled to do such things, myself among them. It follows from the unreasonable nature of an ultramarathon that the ultrarunner's motive must reside in a domain outside reason: the unconscious mind, the shadows of times forgotten, yet still felt.

Life is movement. Even a leaf can turn toward the sun. As a child, I loved to read about the stars and planets. I knew they ran around in loops, driven by fundamental forces of physical being, like clock hands turning on a clockface. Matter isn't free. Planets don't get to choose their orbits. But people do. I do.

Runners: You can see us on the street. You can see us on trails and tracks and sidewalks. Bodies surge forth, arms like pistons, feet kicking the ground, every push-off propelling our hard, sinuous limbs in hyperkinetic leaps that accelerate with every revolution—the movement of liberation.

But there is another kind of runner. See the frightened ones, crouched in the alleys and doorways, faces wan and haggard. Perhaps you wonder where they came from, or what rage or madness brought them there, these wounded souls. Exiles. Runaways.

Runners and runaways: life moves between these two poles of possibility, between what you choose and what gets chosen for you. One exists in conscious motion; the other follows an unbidden path on an orbit set forth by history or the structure of reality. The runner picks a point a hundred meters or a hundred miles away and decides to move toward it. The runaway feels the impulse in the background, the momentum upon which physics or history threw you into being, from the spiral loops of the galaxies and the orbit of Earth to the life cycles of cells in your body and the legacies of love and hate that loop across generations and centuries. To be human is to be a composite of both kinds of revolving cycles: conscious yet unconscious, a spirit at once free and determined, a rhythm between earth and air, like feet leaving the ground and then landing again. I understand both kinds of running because I have lived them. I am a runaway who became a runner, a trauma survivor who became a trauma psychologist and an ultramarathoner.

Two hundred miles: what an ordeal of such dimensions would do to my body and mind, I wasn't certain. But I had an inkling. I'd been running vast distances for years. I had run in the blazing heat of the desert and across the Grand Canyon. I had run a hundred seventy miles of the John Muir Trail in five days and nonstop for thirty hours in the Wasatch Mountains of Utah until my feet turned into a bloody mess. Run far enough and things fall apart. The center cannot hold. Total anarchy is loosed upon the mind. In that state of breakdown, it's sometimes hard for me to remember why running all day and night through the mountains ever seemed like a good idea. *When I get done with this madness*, I think, *I'm never coming back. This is the last time.*

But it never is. Twenty hours into a run, alone in the dark, marching uphill through the forest, the finish line might as well be a million miles away. In that state of dejection, I can even find it hard to believe that the sun will ever rise again. The darkness feels all too familiar. Now and then I see others on the trail, their weary faces glowing in my headlamp with the spectral pallor of revenants, tired souls wandering in exile from some forgotten disaster, yearning to be led to rest.

Then something happens in the sunrise. The dark horizon turns into azure. I feel the warmth on my face. All the color comes back in the world and I sense something inside me transform as the path ahead becomes luminous and the leaves wave at me in the golden dawn like a million little hands: *Welcome back to life.* The feeling that soaks through me when the darkness transforms into claps, whoops, and the clang of a faraway bell is something like resurrection.

In the dawn, remembering the night's dejection, I have an intuition that the darkness must have *meant something*: the cold and silence and endless trudging through the forest was all too familiar. But like the fragments of a half-remembered dream that fades upon waking, the meaning gets left behind in the dark. And that is the answer to my daughter's question. I need to go back into the darkness. I need to hear the message in the darkness. I need to remember.

MIDWAY ALONG THE WESTERN shore of Lake Tahoe is a ski resort called Homewood. The circular course of the Tahoe 200 starts and finishes there. I arrived at Homewood around noon yesterday. Inside the ski lodge an intrepid young woman in a trucker hat—Candice, the race director—sat behind a table at the front of the room with satellite images of the course on the projection screen above her. She and her young male colleague beside her then narrated every twist and turn and 40,000 cumulative feet of climbing over the 200 miles of our circumambulation around the lake. To be precise, the course is 205.5 miles. At mile 200, those final 5 miles will seem like another 200. I listened to the race director and her colleague as I stood in line for my medical evaluation. I remembered how when I started running trails a decade earlier I struggled to run for a whole hour, and this run *took an hour to describe*. I tried to remember all the details. I might as well have tried to remember a thousand digits of pi. I let my mind drift.

I got chatting with a runner from Connecticut called Chris and a runner from Belize called Don. "There are a whole bunch of folks here from Connecticut," said Chris. The coincidence struck all three of us as meaningful. The meaning itself eluded articulation. Don told me about the new trekking poles he was using. He had the poles in his hands. I admired their sturdiness. I knew almost nothing about these men, Chris from Connecticut and Don from Belize. Yet already they felt like brothers.

I reached the front of the line. I sat down. A young woman with long brown hair and kind eyes introduced herself as Angel. She was a nurse practitioner, she said. She was the medical director. I understood that as a practitioner of the healing arts she had taken a vow to protect the living. To do no harm. And yet she understood that we ultrarunners are compelled to hurt ourselves as a hobby. She would indulge this strange passion, she said. But she wouldn't let us die.

Angel took my wrist in her hand to measure my resting heart rate. It was normal. She wrapped a cuff around my arm to evaluate my blood pressure. It too was normal. What a comfort it can be to learn that one is normal. "Have we met before?" she said. "Perhaps in Moab?"

"I don't think so," I said. We didn't know each other. And yet I felt that we might have. Not that we had actually ever met or knew each other. But for a second, a dreamlike kind of space had formed between us, in which I could sense an aura of mutual recognition.

"Ever run a two-hundred-miler before?" she said.

"No," I said. "Just a one-hundred. Four times."

"A two-hundred's a different animal," she said. "You have to sleep. Even just an hour every night. That'll make the difference between thinking straight and totally losing it. If you start to hallucinate, lie down and take a nap. It doesn't matter where you are. Even way out in the middle of the wilderness."

"Will do," I said, counting myself a lucky fellow indeed to receive a lesson about sleeping and insanity from this Angel.

At about 8:45 the next morning I saw the pack assembling at the start line. The race director called us to attention. "Repeat after me," she said. "If I get lost or die . . ." *If I get lost or die*, everyone repeated. ". . . it's my own damn fault." *It's my own damn fault.* I closed my eyes. I held my hands in prayer. I remembered what my Zen teacher, Shosan, had told me. I remembered my intention for the run. *Namu kie Butsu*, I said to myself: *I take refuge in the Buddha. In the possibility of awakening. The possibility of liberation.* Then I heard a countdown from ten to zero and started running. One step forward. Half a million to go.

The trail led from the lakeshore up a grassy bank and into the trees. I settled right away into the kind of easy rhythm that, given enough snacks and a catnap here and there, I could maintain forever. The leaders charged uphill and vanished into the forest. One was a former United

States Marine, another perhaps the toughest female trail runner in the world. She once ran 238 miles in the desert and won the race outright, beating the fastest male by ten hours. Another time she ran until she went blind. It occurred to me that her journey as a runner was in that sense the mirror image of my own. I started running afflicted by a kind of blindness. I ran until I could see.

I made no attempt to chase either one of the leaders: *Godspeed, warriors.* I counted myself fortunate to be living and strong enough to relish the long hours of joy and pain on the trail. I didn't need to be the fastest. I didn't care about my time. I cared about time, about memory, about the way long hours on a trail seem to open hidden doors to a dimension of consciousness where present and past become one.

As the pack of runners spread out, I observed the spaces that likewise emerged in between my thoughts. At first my thoughts jostled together for position, jittery with the nervous excitement of a huge experience imagined for months as an approaching horizon, like a faraway mountain of the mind. But then they settled into a calmer rhythm, opening gaps between them. The spaces filled with sensation and emotion, with the sunlit woods and the smell of fir trees and sunscreen and the feeling of strength in my legs, with the joy of being alive and moving on the ground. I had nothing to worry about. Nothing to think about. Nothing I needed to do except grip my left pole and plant it in the dirt a couple of feet ahead, drive my right foot into the trail behind me, push off and swing the right pole forward, plant the pole as my left foot thrust me forward, feel my breath moving in and out and in again without effort or strain as my thoughts . . . spread . . . out. The trail wound back and forth, rising three thousand vertical feet through the forest. The gaps between runners grew longer. I soon had the trail to myself, relishing a spacious feeling in my mind that stretched as wide as the mountains.

And that's how it's been for the past hour. Once in a while I'll pass another runner, or vice versa, and say hello, but the rest of the time I'm alone in the forest and the free-flowing state of mind that I start to get into after a decent stretch of time on a trail.

I pass a guy standing beside the trail, looking at the view. In almost any other sort of running event, you don't see that many people stopping for more than a minute to snap a photo. That's the kind of running in which most people care about *getting somewhere*. This is different. I could say we've got all day, but that's not quite true. We've got *a hundred hours*. We may as well stop once in a while to smell the wildflowers and look at the view.

Especially when we get a view like this one. It goes on forever, a vast green wilderness stretching about a hundred miles to a line of granite peaks on a remote horizon.

"Is it *all* this amazing?" says my fellow runner. It's his first time in California, he tells me. First time in the Sierra Nevada. *First time in the mountains*. Where he comes from, in the flatlands, the view is fields in every direction. Corn as high as an elephant's eye. Not even a bump in sight from his front door to the horizon.

"Yes," I say. "It really is all this amazing." Every last tree and stream and cloud and stone and sunrise. The kind of magnificence so immense you could stare at it for a hundred lifetimes. Some kinds of joy are so big, everyone on the planet could have their fill and there'd be infinity left over.

"You're in for the most incredible views of your life," I say—which is just as well, I almost think to add, knowing how these crazy mountain adventures tend to go: before long, bliss turns into blisters and awe turns into *Ow*, but you suffer less when you know there's always beauty somewhere around the next corner.

The Things I Carry

Run two hundred miles and you can't think about the whole distance. Run *twenty* miles and you're still better off focusing on the mile you're in. But if you run a lot, twenty becomes the sort of feasible distance you can fit in your head. Get out the door early enough and you'll be done before breakfast. For me, the same feeling of feasibility goes for fifty or even sixty miles, because I'm usually done by dinnertime. Beyond that dinnertime threshold, though, the enormity of the path ahead can start to boggle the mind. You think of regular people going to bed, while you're still running. Sleeping, while you're halfway up some hill, still running. Waking tomorrow morning. And so on. And that's *one hundred* miles, which I've run four times; it takes me about thirty hours. If you think of running distances like arithmetic, you'd assume two hundred miles is twice as hard as a hundred. But the increase in effort as you ramp up the distances isn't arithmetical but exponential. The actual energetic differences are hard to quantify, but in my experience a marathon isn't twice as hard as a half-marathon; it's five times harder. A hundred-mile run isn't four regular marathons end to end; it's the labors of Hercules—a whole lifetime in a day and a half. So heaven only knows what's in store over *two hundred* miles.

If I let my mind wander to how it's going to feel at, say, mile 190, the whole adventure starts to seem impossible. The trick, I've found, is to screen everything past the next ten miles completely out of awareness. So that's what I'm doing now. I'm running through the trees, feeling the warm breeze on my face. If I let my thoughts turn to the future at all, I think about the aid station at mile 10: Stephen Jones, it's called, in honor of a man who finished this run a couple of summers ago and died in an avalanche the following winter. None of us is here for very long.

I'm also reminding myself of my plan. Get to mile 50 by midnight. Sleep for an hour. Get to mile 100 by midnight on day two. Sleep for another couple of hours. That's when Emily joins me. If you go to pieces, it's good to have a doctor around, in my experience. Hence: Emily. Once upon a time she was a professional skier. She competed in that event in which the skiers race for miles cross-country with rifles on their backs. Then she went to one of the top medical schools in the world and aced all her exams and stayed awake for thirty hours straight every week saving people's lives. It's hard to imagine a more competent person to have with me by the time I'm hobbling up some hill on wounded stumps, moaning, *Why?* Emily will run with me until mile 180. That will put me about seventy hours into the race. I'll likely be unraveling a bit mentally by then. That's when Miriam comes in. She is used to seeing me lose it, and I am used to her seeing me in a state of loss. Miriam will be with me until the bitter end, sometime late Monday night or Tuesday morning.

I'M HUNGRY. I GRAB a sugar GU packet from one of the front pockets in my pack, tear it open, and swallow the gel. Salted caramel: not bad.

I choose my GU flavors carefully. I think I can say that I choose everything in my pack with quite a fanatical measure of care. Head out on a really big adventure, and it pays to sweat the small stuff. Last night, after we left the ski lodge and drove a couple of miles to our lodgings, I laid out all my running kit on the bed. I wanted to review my equipment checklist one last time before I set off into the mountains.

Lace up your shoes, grab your house key, and get out the door—any normal sort of running tends to be quite simple. That's one of running's joys. You don't need much of anything. I can run for a couple of hours with nothing on my back but the wind. But beyond that two-hour threshold, I do need to carry a few things. Water. Food. Maybe an extra layer or a raincoat. The more miles, the more stuff. When you're planning a *really* long run, say a hundred miles, you have to keep a few principles in mind. You don't have to be totally self-sufficient, like a climber heading off to the Himalayas. Every few miles you'll reach an aid station, where you can fill up on food and water. During the really long ultras—sixty miles, a hundred miles, even farther—you can leave a bag at some of the aid stations with extra kit like a spare pair of shoes or a headlamp. But the aid stations in long mountain ultras tend to be quite spread out. You might be out on your own in the wilderness for ten or fifteen or even twenty miles, for instance, before you get to the next one. Depending on how steep the trail gets, and how exhausted you are, that can mean being out by yourself for six or eight or even ten hours, in the wind or rain or snow or blazing heat, depending on the part of the country you're in and the time of year. Out in the wilderness solo for any length of time, and you need *stuff.* You want to travel as light as possible—but not *too* light. Is it better to have something and not need it or end up needing something but not have it? That was the question I'd been pondering for the past six months, getting ready for the run. I must have gone through my kit list twenty times to make sure I hadn't forgotten anything. Here's what I laid out on the bed:

1. Shoes, socks, extra socks
2. Shirt, shorts, bandanna, gloves, cap, shades
3. Lightweight carbon-fiber fold-up trekking poles
4. Energy gels and bars
5. GPS tracker, phone, waterproof camera
6. Digital music player (Loaded with tunes appropriate to the full catastrophe of human emotion, from Whitney Houston to Slipknot, for there will surely come a time when I'll feel so blissed out I'll want to sing like Whitney: *"I wanna dance with somebody!"* But doubtless there also will be moments when, in the words of the Slipknot song "Psychosocial," I'll be close to tears on a mountaintop, thinking, *"I did my time, and I want out."*)
7. Hand wipes (I can't stand having sticky hands. I'll put up with almost anything: cramps, diarrhea, blisters, lacerations, illusions, hallucinations, delusions of omnipotence, despair, mosquitoes, bloody

urine, backache, leg ache, knee ache, neck ache, butt ache. But having sticky hands really puts me over the edge.)

8. Twenty dollars in cash, a little laminated card with my address and phone number and emergency contact, photos of my kids, and a lucky bracelet that my daughter made for me

9. Race bib (I'm number 108. The race organizers let us runners choose our own numbers. I like the number 108. It's the number of names of the Divine Mother in Hinduism.)

10. Whistle, compass, knife, waterproof matches, survival blanket (Likely I won't get lost and need this stuff. But better to have it and not need it than the other way around. I've learned that lesson the hard way. Go out into the wilderness and you need to have a plan for when everything goes to shit and you're on your own. You have to assume the non-zero risk of a catastrophic outcome and think through what is required to survive. The survival blanket is a thin golden Mylar sheet folded into a four-inch square. You get cold fast when you're exhausted. Unfold your little golden square, wrap it around you, and it keeps you warm by reflecting your own body heat.)

As runs go, that's quite a lot of stuff. But it all fits in a little twelve-liter purple pack that's so light and fits so nice and snug on my back that I can almost forget it's there.

And even if it's a lot to carry, by running standards, the list of things I *won't* be carrying wouldn't fit on a single page. For that, you'd need a whole book.

Children need parents to keep them safe. The little ones need to know that Mom or Dad is watching. You start out crawling to a toy at the other side of the room; you wind up moving out and starting your own independent adult life. It feels okay to move away from Mom or Dad when you can sense their caring presence behind you, what the psychologist John Bowlby called *attachment*. At the beginning, this feeling of security means literally being held—cradled in a loving parent's arms and knowing your needs are seen and will be taken care of. After feeling held and seen like this, you come to understand yourself as worthy of being held and seen. It's not long until you can walk and then run, and even if Mom and Dad are thousands of miles away, you carry that feeling inside you of being held and seen, like a warmth-reflecting blanket tucked in your backpack.

But some children don't get held and seen when they're little. Mom and Dad don't know how—nobody taught them. You can't remember being held and seen. Or you remember being slapped in the face, seen by eyes with a look that scared you or made no sense at all. You come to expect a life that slaps you in the face. You come to understand yourself as mad or bad or dangerous to know. Exhausted on the trail of life, you may reach for the blanket in your pack, and what it reflects isn't warmth but all the times you cried and nobody was there. Or you get used to stumbling forward past the point of exhaustion because there's no safe way of stopping. Or maybe you look for a better blanket. Compared to the tinfoil variety, a good emotional blanket can be hard to find. There are blankets that look good but turn out not to be. The booze-and-drugs blanket. The toxic-relationship blanket.

To run ahead with confidence as a child means knowing your care-givers see you. This confidence is a type of bodily knowledge, or implicit memory, that shapes a young human's basic sense of being knowable and worthy of attention and care. It is neurologically close to the way you remember how to ride a bike. Imagine not riding a bike for ten years and then picking up a bike and that feeling of your body knowing what to do. Your earliest relationships with caregivers likewise shape a basic sense of your ability to move safely in the world. The word *trauma* comes from the ancient Greek word for *wound*. Bleeding defines the most obvious kinds of injury, but a less visible form cuts deeper: the enduring effects on the mind, body, and nervous system caused by a lack of dependable emotional nurturing in your earliest relationships with primary care-givers, called *attachment trauma*. Unsafe and unseen children become runaways. After you start running, it's hard to believe that it's safe to stop, hard to trust that the danger is really behind you.

The unwritten manual of the human species lists certain items essential to survival. You need a good survival blanket—something or someone that reflects warmth and love and caring, a blanket you can crawl under a tree with in the depth of night and wrap around you until the sun comes, a way to feel held and seen and to believe that you deserve to survive.

II

Mercury

Dreaming

From the high country, the trail descends two thousand feet through the trees. I love running fast downhill. Build up the leg strength to handle the pounding, let gravity do its work, and soon you're falling through space with the wind in your face and the feeling of bliss that comes along with everything rushing at you, the trail and the trees and this turn to the left and now a turn to the right, the rhythm of the ground coming up to meet your feet and then falling away again. The faster you go, the more time in the air. Run fast enough and you can almost imagine leaving the ground altogether and soaring like a bird in the sky above. I love the feeling so much, I'm tempted to let it rip: lean forward, hammer the ground, prepare for takeoff.

But that would be a mistake. On a twenty-mile run, sure—have at it. Even on a fifty-mile run. Worst case, I roll an ankle or trip and hit the dirt and get scratched up a bit. And no doubt my leg muscles would feel a bit sore in the morning. But on a two-hundred-miler? No. I think of my muscles and tendons and ligaments as a family on an epic road trip. There's a limit to how much the little ones can handle. If I'm nice and gentle now, later on, when everyone's totally exhausted, I'll still have a decent shot at keeping the whole crew somewhat together, instead of having everyone break down yelling and sobbing and screaming and saying, *Please won't you stop that, really. I'm begging you, please.*

..

The garden covered a third of an acre. It might as well have been a country. In the autumn the lawn became a blanket of leaves, which my brother, Sebastian, and I raked into piles. We loaded the leaf piles into the wheelbarrow and rolled the barrow down to the compost heap, just beyond the line of fir trees at the bottom of the garden. To step into the trees was to enter another world, a little patch of wilderness. We called it the Jungle. It was a tangle of branches and overgrown weeds. Under the tree canopy, as we crouched through the thicket, everything looked dark green and shadowy. This hidden world existed within the rectangle formed by the line of fir trees and the neighbors' fences. It can't have covered more than a couple hundred square feet. It felt like infinity. Sebastian and I could lose ourselves there for hours. It reminded us of a picture of a forest that once we had seen in a storybook. At midnight, under a full moon, cats came out of their homes and gathered in the forest. The cats linked paws and danced around in a circle. Lying in our beds after our mother tucked us in, we would picture our own cat, a thirty-pound black-and-white tom called Briar, joining all the cats of the neighborhood in the Jungle, dancing in secret under moonlight, long after we both fell asleep. It didn't seem impossible. Almost anything seemed possible in the Jungle.

One time I was exploring the thicket underneath the compost heap when I heard the sound of breathing. I wriggled deeper inside the thicket to follow the breathing sound to its source. It was a hedgehog! I looked at its tiny nose and mouth and eyes. Its body got a little bigger every time it inhaled, and then smaller again as it exhaled. With each exhale, it let out a little sigh. "Sebastian, you have to get in here," I said. I wriggled out of the thicket. Sebastian went inside to see.

Soon it was getting dark. It was almost time for supper. We would need to leave the Jungle and walk back up through the garden to the house. If we were lucky, Mummy would make us chocolate fudge pudding for dessert. Perhaps we would tell Mummy and Daddy about the hedgehog, we thought. But it would be hard to explain the feeling. We could go on talking until the end of time, telling them how it felt, two little boys together seeing something otherworldly in the undergrowth, but nobody else could ever really know the hidden world Sebastian and

I knew, the feeling of a mystery glimpsed only by us, deep in the trees, before the light began to fade and we went indoors for the night.

..

Running is powerful medicine for the mind. Put on your shoes and run down the trail or sidewalk and something shifts on the inside. A feeling of mellow euphoria soaks through you as the brain releases natural chemicals called endocannabinoids. Your mind feels clearer. Sharper. But run far enough and the mind soon shifts from euphoria into a kind of waking dream state.

A person is a fusion of two beings: reasoner and dreamer. The reasoner can think and plan and remember. The dreamer can wonder and create. Run down a steep, rocky trail and you have to focus. *See that hole: land on the other side of it.* Your body works hard to keep you upright and moving. Sweat cools you down. A lot of these things carry on in the background. Run for an hour and your brain goes about business as usual. But run all day and your brain senses some sort of disaster occurring. Automatic mechanisms switch on in deep brain regions, hardwired by millions of years of evolution to make sure you survive. You need to swallow and pee and keep on moving. The thinking parts of your brain go quiet. Psychologist Arne Dietrich coined the term *transient hypofrontality* for this phenomenon.[2] *Hypo* means *under*, as in *underactive*. *Frontality* refers to the prefrontal cortex, the part of the brain that supports higher cognitive functions like memory and reason.

Lucky for you this holiday from thinking doesn't last forever. Lose some functionality of your prefrontal cortex and it tends to get tricky to, say, find your car keys. Imagine losing it all, waking one morning not knowing who you are or even *what* you are. You would be in hell.

It turns out there are gentler ways to turn off all that thinking. One of them you know well. It's the place your mind runs free at night: the dreamworld. Your dreaming mind stitches together a crazy story from random memory fragments as it runs wherever it wants to, through the traces of everything you've ever thought and felt, all the way back to the womb, perhaps to the origin of the species and ancient evolutionary time. You wake up and your mind feels clearer.

But sometimes you can't sleep, or your dreams are terrifying nightmares. I used to have a recurring dream in which I was being chased. I tried to run, but my legs couldn't move, like I was held in place by some invisible force. Without the ability to dream, the mind starts getting messy, like a dense forest where all the trails are overgrown. Today feels like yesterday, or last year.

There are different kinds of dreams. There are night dreams and daydreams and times when reality goes dreamy and unreal because you're blissed out or scared. There are many trails back to the dreamworld. Humanity has mapped that psychic trail system since the dawn of time. There are trance dances. There are pilgrimages. There are psychedelic drug states. And there are runs in the mountains that go on for days and nights.

When I run, my body leaves the ground for a moment but then comes back down again, a cycle between earth and air, gravity and flight, the terrestrial and the heavenly. With my every step, Earth says, *I am here.* So that's what I'm looking forward to these days and nights ahead of me on the trail. Not thinking. Dreaming.

Hear the Clock Tick-Tock

I chased the firefighter inside the smoking tower block and followed him sprinting up the spiral stairwell. I could hear him panting with the hard effort in his blue woolen suit and black plastic helmet as I matched his pace step for step, propelled by the energy of a fit twenty-eight-year-old in ripped jeans and a yellow sleeveless soccer shirt with nothing to lose. At around the sixth flight of stairs he glanced back at me, and I registered the surprise in his eyes as he saw that I was still behind him. I followed him through a door from the stairwell to the top-floor lobby. Smoke billowed from the open door of one of the apartments. He took three deep breaths, held the last one in, and strode into the apartment.

It was the spring of 1999. Two decades before the Tahoe 200, I was in Mumbai, India, working as a documentary researcher for British television. I spent my days in Mumbai talking to Bollywood action movie stars and one-limbed beggars and a cabdriver who had come to the city as a runaway five-year-old orphan from a village hundreds of miles away and had a huge distended belly from what he understood was cancer and who drove around in his yellow cab with a sign on the back that said DON'T FORGET GOD AND DEATH and in the sunset stood by the brown polluted waters near the fancy hotels at Nariman Point drinking whiskey, a bottle every night, which he split with me, fifty-fifty.

In the evenings I ran through the 100-degree heat, inhaling the humid air fragrant with sandalwood and sewage, rivers of sweat pouring from my face and chest, dodging cars and skinny cows and throngs of little emaciated homeless children in rags staring at me with their sad eyes, saying, "Please, sir. Please, jogger man. One rupee, sir," and then at night I would take a rickshaw to Nariman Point Fire Station and lie in bed, still with my clothes on, my camera on the floor right next to me, waiting for the siren. The station chief was a local legend, the bravest firefighter in Mumbai, or perhaps the world. An article I had read about him in one of the papers reported his actions in the aftermath of a terrorist bomb about a decade earlier that had blown up the Bombay Stock Exchange. Prabhat had been first on the scene. The Mumbai Fire Brigade fought fires wearing woolen suits and a smattering of rusty breathing apparatuses that resembled nineteenth-century diving kit. Prabhat had run into the ruins of the building to search for survivors, ignoring warnings from colleagues that the terrorists might have lain booby traps inside. He was the purest archetype of heroism I could possibly imagine. Yet he wore his bravery with the humble air of a quiet and jolly man, with a hearty laugh, who doted on his wife and daughter and understood his heroic actions as the choiceless outcome of the role that the secret and sacred cycles of the universe had bestowed upon him. "It is my karma," he said, and he picked up his smiling daughter, put her on his knee, and giggled with her, then looked toward me, asking me why I always looked so serious.

It was dark in the corridor that led from the apartment's doorway to the inferno in the living room. The thick black smoke stung my eyes. I pointed my camera at the firefighter. Holding my breath, I figured I had about ninety seconds before I'd need to get out. The blaze in the living room through the smoke-shrouded camera lens appeared as a blurry orange flicker in the upper fifth of the dark frame. I crept farther into the living room. The fierce heat of the air seared the skin on my face and forearms. The firefighter glanced behind him and saw me. "Get out!" he yelled. "Get out now!" I held my shot of the firefighter for a couple of seconds longer and then ran back out of the room.

I had to keep running. It was hard to recall a time when I hadn't needed to run, to chase one mad adventure after another. By the late '90s, I had a job as a freelance television documentary producer in London. The work could take me almost anywhere. I could have picked less dangerous assignments—a gardening show, for instance. In a forgotten eon I might have felt happy in a garden. But not anymore. Stay in one place, in the same room, relationship, job, city, or even continent, and the Darkness caught up with me: a sad, worried, desperate, trapped feeling that had lurked inside me as long as I could remember, and got worse the longer I remained motionless. If I kept moving, I stayed ahead of the Darkness. I felt like Dr. David Bruce Banner in *The Incredible Hulk* TV show I had watched as a kid.

You know the story. At the start, he's this regular guy. He shows up someplace random, where no one knows him, looking for a fresh start. *Hi, I'm David*, he says. *I'm looking for work. No, you can't be my friend, because you won't like me when I'm angry.* Then disaster strikes! A landslide. A plane crash. Now David is angry. His muscles blow up five times their regular size. His shirt rips open. He has this mad look in his eyes. Now you've done it: *Goodbye, mild-mannered David. Hello, Hulk.* He saves everyone. Afterward, they can't wait to thank the strange green monster who came to their rescue. But now his secret is out! How dearly regular old David yearns to stay, finally settle someplace where people really know him, someplace where he belongs. But there's that pesky gumshoe reporter on his heels. *Who is this so-called Hulk? The public has a right to know . . .* David's gotta go. As the credits roll, there he is again, week after week, hiking at the edge of town, knapsack over his shoulder, hitching a ride to next week's identical episode.

That was me. On the outside I wore the mask of a mild-mannered English nerd. But find out the secret horrors that lurked deep within me, and you wouldn't like what you saw.

I spent six months in Mumbai. When the day drew near for my return trip to London, I wondered, *What's next?* I could picture myself in my dingy flat, sitting at my desk, waiting for the phone to ring. I took a rickshaw through the boiling heat to an internet café. There was no such thing as a smartphone in those days. The internet was a simpler and far less insane place, composed, for the most part, of words and photos and perhaps a dozen grainy cat videos. Sweat dripped from my face as I entered the air-conditioned interior of the café. I sat down at one of the computers. I clicked the mouse to open Internet Explorer. I typed in the address for some crazy festival in the Nevada desert that my old college friend Ned and I had talked about going to in the early fall. Our friend Robin had been to it the year before. Burning Man was utterly bonkers, she said. You could do and be absolutely anything you wanted there. People gave everything away for free. Some of the participants had worked for months or even years on insane sculptures, like dragons that breathed actual fire. Show up in the desert and wander around at random and you saw miracles in every direction. At the end, they burned a giant effigy of a man, and after you had danced all night for days, high on drugs, something burned up inside you as well, and so you went home feeling as if the fire that engulfed the giant Man had also burned up all the old rubbish in your mind.

I completed my assignment in Mumbai. I flew back to London. Among the junk mail and postcards from my mother on the stack of mail my flatmate had left on my desk, I found an envelope postmarked from San Francisco, California, containing a ticket with a warning printed on the back: YOU VOLUNTARILY ASSUME THE RISK OF SERIOUS DEATH OR INJURY BY ATTENDING THIS EVENT. *Sounds like just my sort of thing*, I thought.

FROM SAN FRANCISCO, I drove east with Ned and Robin via the shimmering casinos of Reno and about a hundred miles north into a flat, white high desert that stretched to mountains in the far distance beneath the limitless azure sky that formed a featureless plane of vaster dimension than I had ever encountered anywhere on Earth. Nothing much had happened here since the Pleistocene, and to inhabit its primordial aura catalyzed a perceptual shift into geologic time.

The camps were positioned in a series of concentric circles that formed an enormous U-shaped array, enclosing the empty expanse of desert, at the center of which stood the giant Man. The concentric circles were organized in a plan that duplicated the Copernican model of the solar system. The closest circle to the center was named Mercury; radiating outward were Venus, Earth, Mars, Jupiter, Saturn, Uranus, and Neptune. Radial streets, numbered 2:00 through 10:00, intersected the circles like the hour positions on a clock. According to the event guide, which I had read on the internet, the theme that year was The Wheel of Time. As I gazed across the expanse of the desert and the vast blue sky above, anything seemed possible. I put glitter on my chest and rabbit ears on my head. Ned put on a top hat and an orange sarong and daubed his face and bare upper body with blue body paint so to me he wound up looking something like the English-toff equivalent of Krishna. I opened the van door and stepped onto the dusty ground. A warm wind blew in my face. Techno thundered *oontz* in the distance. The low evening sun cast long shadows of the people crossing the white plain on bicycles and bathed everything in a golden light. Our wandering path through the desert brought us to a man with several large and expensive-looking cameras draped around his neck. "Can I take your picture?" he said, looking at Ned. *Why not mine?* I thought. I watched the photographer snap several pictures of Ned in different poses from multiple angles, switching from one big camera to an even bigger one with a long lens for a close-up. "Good luck finding your party, Bunny Man," the photographer said. I felt diminished in his eyes. Yet I soon came to appreciate the giant scale of psychedelic marvels against which a humble rabbit disappeared in the dust clouds.

In every direction I saw something unprecedented and magical. A tree made of bones. A buried submarine, its prow emerging from the dust. Wandering farther, I encountered a wooden box upon whose sides were inscribed the words *hope, wish, prayer, dream*—the creation, I discovered later, of an artist called Steven Raspa—and from which a woman's voice emerged to utter prophecies. "In the future," said the prophetess, "we will remember the peacefulness of parking lots . . . Everyone will receive a single orange ticket . . . Children will scrape their knees on the sound barrier . . ."

I approached a scaffold structure above which hung a sign that said CAMP DOS. I understood the name as an allusion to the acronym for *disc operating system*. I learned that no such technological meaning was intended. The name invoked the Spanish *dos*: Camp Two. But two of what? No one knew.

I drank a pint-size margarita as the sun sank close to the horizon, and Ned and I washed down our Ecstasy pills with swigs of orange Gatorade and waited for nightfall. All my fear was gone. I was aware of needing to breathe out with slow, heavy sighs to steady the crashing waves on the inside that shifted now into delicious electric tingles shooting up and down my spine. I walked toward the music and the pulsing green and orange lasers. I began to move in time with the bass and the shimmer of the lights and with the bodies moving next to mine, all the people with their smiling faces and eyes that when they saw me did not look away but rather held me in the single field of light into which all our gazes merged as one, and I felt my body moving with the boom and pulse and with every man and woman as if it were our bodies moving together that made the music and the light.

The camps shone in kaleidoscopic fluorescents. A man in a fire-protective suit standing on a truck fired lightning bolts from a device in his arm, launching the bolts high above his head with a shrieking sound. A circus troupe appeared, juggling sticks on fire. I saw Ned's pupils dilate in drugged wonder. A tingling sensation shot from my lumbar vertebrae to the base of my skull. "Oh my God," I said, breathing hard, like I'd just run a fifty-meter dash, as waves of pleasure rippled from my sacrum and up my back. I felt an inner weight lift from me, as if conferring a reprieve from an ancient and forgotten crime. I was aware of the pounding techno and the flashing lights converging into a kind of single living field of warmth that beckoned me to merge with it. A glittery dome appeared in the distance and I walked toward it as if drawn to the tunnel of light reported in near-death experiences. Time dissolved into a single radiant now as I wandered to one distant shimmer far away and then back across the desert to another. I encountered a woman in a silver gown with whom I fell into conversation concerning children's television. We could both remember the names of all four Teletubbies and repeated them in unison. Tinky Winky. Dipsy. Laa-Laa. Po. Her blue eyes met mine and did not look away.

As the sky turned from black to cobalt, I returned to our van and fell asleep for a while. The square of blue sky I saw through the van window in the dawn filled me with an inexplicable sadness. I became conscious of my impending departure. I could picture the gray skies of London and could feel the futility that would creep through my veins as I walked through the city streets alone in the cold, damp darkness of the long English winter. I wandered with mild despair through a waking dreamworld, an environment created by the sort of unrepressed human beings I had always imagined might exist somewhere in the world but seldom encountered in England. I was conscious of the beauty and freedom outside me and of my role as observer. I took my clothes off and covered my body in red paint and put my bunny ears back on and ran through the desert.

As the sun sank low again in the sky, I climbed the scaffold of Camp Dos to eat dinner while watching the sun set. Afterward, I descended the scaffold by a ladder with a salad bowl in my left hand, holding the ladder with my right. A woman observed my awkward descent and took the salad bowl out of my hand to help me. I thanked her and then went into the van to dress for the evening. I joined a crowd of thousands assembled in a circle around the wooden effigy of a man with his arms held aloft like a runner first across the finish line. A long time passed. "Will someone please burn this fucking man before our drugs wear off," someone said, to laughter. The scale of the inferno that soon engulfed the Man transcended any fire I had previously witnessed. A swirl of orange spirals wrapped together and morphed like something alive and sentient, its tangerine glow igniting the crowd into yawps and whistles.

The inferno reminded me of Guy Fawkes Night. I remembered how the name of the park in the middle of town where the bonfire took place every year in my youth was mysterious because I heard the word *arbor* as an abbreviation of *harbor*. The park thus had fused in my mind with a cryptic resonance of the maritime, as if haunted by ghost ships. In the Arbor in October the people of our little town left offerings of rubbish: branches of dead and dying trees; broken chairs and tables; clothes; newspapers and even unwanted books. Day after day, the pile of rubbish grew, until the stack rose twenty-five or thirty feet high, a pyramid of debris in the center of the park, and then on the fifth of November they lit it on fire. The streets were full of people, and we made our way toward the Arbor carrying sparklers, chatting, and laughing, craning our necks as we heard the whoosh of rockets blossoming in the dark sky like magic flowers. The air smelled of gunpowder, and we were eager to reach the Arbor, but there was no way of moving faster than the crowd itself, so we gave ourselves to this movement, and soon we had flowed into the park, past the stalls illuminated in pink and purple neon. I was struck by the fire's heat on my face, even from fifty yards. Pressed against the metal railing, gripping Mummy's hand, I was amazed by the fire's power, by a heat so intense I could not face it directly for more than a few seconds. Later, we watched the bright spinning Catherine wheels and more rockets soaring high above us, but it was the bonfire that commanded my fascination even as the crowd began to dissipate, leaving small groups of teenagers with plastic bottles of cider. For others, it was a fire that commemorated the defeat of Catholic insurrection in the ritual immolation of a traitor's effigy, but knowledge of gunpowder treason was lost to me, for the figure I saw in the flames was not Guy Fawkes but the captain of the 'arbor—a sailor shouting, *Ahoy, ahoy there, ahoy.*

The Man burned. I did more Ecstasy and danced until the morning. From the Black Rock Desert on the drive back west to San Francisco, Ned, Robin, and I stopped for the night at a motel on the north shore of Lake Tahoe. Several Camp Dos members were also staying there en route to Bay Area homes. Before dinner at a Mexican restaurant, we gathered in one of the motel rooms. Everyone was showered and groomed and, absent the dust and glitter and costumes, hard to recognize. I sat down on one of the beds. "Hi, I'm Miriam," said the woman on the bed opposite me. I was conscious of her beauty and of her kind eyes looking at me. Over dinner, along with tacos and margaritas, we shared shards of memory. I felt as if we had all woken from a collective crazy dream, shattered in a million random story fragments about dragons and trees made of bones and buried submarines. Sometimes one person's piece of the dream fit with a piece owned by someone else, so the two of them could put the pieces together in a form that corroborated the existence of dragons and bone trees in the desert. But other times, all that could be recalled from the dreamworld in its aftermath was a solo mad wander through the dust storm, and the uncanny convergence of impossible things that appeared when the wanderer was lost there. Such singular memory fragments belonged to the wanderer alone. Everyone remembered Dr. Megavolt: the man atop a truck in a protective fire suit with a gizmo strapped to his arm; the crackle of lightning, audible from half a mile away, as the air fizzed with millions of volts and Megavolt raised his arm and a cobalt fork of lightning shot from the gizmo, igniting the crowd beneath this modern Prometheus in uproar; the hallucinatory perception, as we stood beneath him, that perhaps we had been transported to a distant future era in which humans had become godlike beings who could channel universal forces with the power of their minds.

To Miriam, she told me later, I seemed extremely serious, an Englishman in glasses droning on about Prometheus, until in passing I disclosed my rabbit alter ego. These two identities struck her as surprising in their coexistence. In turn, I realized that the woman who had known the Teletubbies and the woman who had helped me down from the scaffold were one and the same: this Miriam. Long ago, when people looked at the horizon, they saw two lights, one at dawn and the other in the evening. They called the first one the morning star. They called the second one the evening star. In time they learned that the two lights were in reality a single one, shining not from stars but from a sphere much closer to Earth, Venus, the planet named after the goddess of love. The two women from Camp Dos were in reality a single Miriam: she was lovely.

I completed the journey with Ned back to San Francisco, intending to fly the next day back to London. A plan had emerged for a Camp Dos farewell shindig, to be convened in a nightclub. The campers assembled beforehand in someone's house. I saw Miriam the moment I entered the living room. I was conscious again of her large blue eyes. We said hello. I learned that she was an artist. She sustained her attention upon me as I spoke. I felt liberated in her presence to tell her anything that came to mind, without fearing the sardonic tone that had pervaded almost every conversation in my twenty-nine years in England. I told her about something I'd heard on a record by Fila Brazillia called *Old Codes, New Chaos* that sampled the audio of a journalist describing the LSD experiments performed by the Pentagon on US soldiers in the 1960s. Under the influence of psychedelics, one of the soldiers said he had traveled back in time. It felt important to me that Miriam should know this, significant that she permitted me to tell her about it at some length without interruption, yielding then in her attention upon me the feeling of a force field that pulled our twin gazes into a single timeless zone. We went to the nightclub. I danced with Miriam. We left the club and stood outside on the street. We were standing very close to each other. I took my glasses off. Our lips met. I closed my eyes. The universe collapsed into my consciousness of only the flowing motion of our tongues, a warm, wet darkness within which I felt as if I had always been enclosed.

My announcement in England that I intended to emigrate provoked a lukewarm reaction. I told everyone, even my bank manager. After a decade in which I'd run from one mad adventure to the next, I can imagine this latest departure didn't seem any different. They heard my story about a modern Prometheus in the Nevada desert and the beautiful artist I'd met there after running about naked with bunny ears, and I could imagine them thinking, *Sure, Jason. Move to California. See you in a couple of weeks.* But this time was different, I thought. I could go live with Miriam and at last settle down, I thought. *I won't need to keep on running.*

I WALKED THROUGH CUSTOMS to baggage claim in San Francisco International Airport, listening to a recorded message on the loud-speakers overhead. "Hi, I'm Willie Brown, mayor of San Francisco. Welcome to the City of Lights, the City of *Dee*-lights." I showed my passport to the immigration officer and walked into the arrivals area. I saw Miriam at once, her smile and luminous blue eyes beaming like a beacon. We kissed for quite a while. The road from the airport led to the freeway heading north. I gazed at the bright blue sky above us as she drove us to a street in the middle of the city.

The weather was weird in San Francisco. It was boiling hot in December and freezing cold in July. The rest of the year was an everlasting springtime. I missed how back in England green leaves went brown in the autumn. Every second car in San Francisco had a bumper sticker that said: I'D RATHER BE HERE NOW. Be Here Now was the Californian religion. But where was this place, Now? The more I tried to Be Here Now, the more my thoughts drifted to Back Then. Time was the most elusive runaway of all.

I found work forty-eight hours after landing in California, for a fledgling internet video company. It was the height of the dot-com boom. Well-paid work was plentiful. One day everyone on Earth will be making movies on the internet, the company founder said. His vision seemed to me preposterous and utopian. Yet it also seemed to me that work had always meant my assent to credence in another person's fantasy. I took the job.

Everything has changed, I thought. I was tired of the past. Tired of always rushing toward the horizon, arriving in some faraway airport to see the row of taxi drivers, standing with their signs listing names of arriving travelers, and imagining what might happen if I were to announce myself as Jeremy Jones or Mohammed Iqbal or François Lejeune and follow a random cabdriver to where random chance might take me. But that was back then, in the days of running and madness, before the Man burned and I met Miriam. Here and Now, beneath the blue skies of San Francisco, the Darkness was at last behind me, and ahead I saw nothing but the boundless future.

I STOOD BENEATH a shiny disco ball on a crowded dance floor two weeks later as the music stopped and the DJ began the countdown to midnight. Miriam too stood in the kaleidoscopic light, which cast her white feathered diaphanous gown and her cheeks speckled with silver glitter in a luminous circle. I held her close and looked into her turquoise eyes. *Ten . . . nine . . . eight . . .* All the freaks and dot-commers and Goths and ravers shimmering in fluorescent greens and purples chanted the descending digits in unison with tens of millions assembled in clubs and bars and streets and living rooms up and down the West Coast as something massive and without precedent surged from just beyond the horizon of existence toward becoming now. We could feel it, the energy gathering in the sounds of the whoops and whistles and in the knowledge of an entire epoch coming to an end, the millennium that had stretched from Magna Carta to Henry VIII to Auschwitz to Hiroshima to the moon landing to the invention of the web: the world stood at the threshold of another age. Perhaps it was the end of time. The papers and TV news shows had been full of warnings that all the computers in the world might fail at the stroke of midnight when the clocks designed for double-digit years clicked to zero and sent circuits running haywire. The consequences of clocks going back to a zero hour and crashing all the hard drives in the world at once were unknowable and conceivably apocalyptic: planes might even fall out of the sky.

Seven . . . six . . . five . . . But perhaps the time to come would be one not of disaster but of hope and healing and things brought into being that once we had only dreamed of. A future Earth where six billion human minds joined together in a single World Wide Web: imagine the possibilities! A future where all the rage and darkness of the world in the time before would fade into memory. *Four . . . three . . . two . . .* Our lips came together as one.

My first few months with Miriam were blissful. The sky was blue and cloudless, and I felt sunshine in my soul. Some months later we were sitting on a beach when a feeling of great bliss and wonder overcame me. *I just turned thirty. I live in California. I'm drinking a chocolate milkshake by the Pacific Ocean with my lovely American girlfriend. How did I get this lucky?*

We danced all night. We went running in the woods. We ate delicious cheeses. Sometimes I had little moments of an old, familiar sadness. But the feeling never stuck around. I could always find some new adventure to dive into. And I could always count on Miriam to make me feel better on lazy Sunday afternoons, lying in the park, when my sadness returned. The following autumn, we got married. Among the vows we exchanged, Miriam said, "I promise to stroke your back when you're feeling blue."

Everything had indeed changed: almost the entirety of my waking existence. A new apartment. A new job. Even the plumbing was different. Sometimes the onslaught of novelty was overwhelming. I flooded the bathroom. I took a bite of Chinese takeout that was spicier than I'd anticipated, and I felt like bursting into tears. The internet video company ran into financial troubles after the collapse of the internet bubble. I found work as a reporter for a technology magazine. I had thought I could migrate from England to the US without much ado. I spoke the primary language, after all. But like a plant uprooted from a known environment and set down in foreign soil, I suffered the shock of transplantation. It wasn't so much any single place or person or experience back in England that I could identify as missing so much as a billion little familiar details put together, the whole ground of landscape and culture and identity I'd grown up in, much of it taken for granted. There is only a certain amount of chaos the nervous system can handle. I began to crave the comfort of the familiar. For a while, I ate nothing but bagels and cream cheese. I ran the same three-mile loop around my neighborhood. One day my knee hurt. I didn't know how to take care of it. I gave up running and went surfing instead. It didn't seem like a big deal at the time. I'd been a runner since the chaos of my teens. Running had been the one constant through fifteen years of change, like a quiet friend who never asked for anything but was always there when I needed them.

I WAS STILL HALF-ASLEEP when I heard something on the morning radio news about an explosion in a tower. I thought I was hearing anniversary coverage about the bomb in the '90s. A feeling of apocalyptic dread seized me when I turned on the television and watched a second plane hit the South Tower. The feeling had the ancient quality of a nightmare long suppressed, now crashing back into consciousness. Miriam and I spent the remainder of the morning watching looped television news footage of the towers collapsing as we struggled to integrate the knowledge of an event so big it warped the time around it, fracturing history into the world before the planes hit and the new and frightening time after. I would never again see a jet in a blue sky without picturing a plane flying low above Manhattan and the blue turning into darkness. I heard a story around that time that the dust on people's faces at Ground Zero came from obliterated rocks once mined in or near the Black Rock Desert, that it was the same dust that covered our faces at Burning Man. Whether or not the story was veridical, it expressed a kind of truth: the psychological need in those fearful days to build new links between the broken fragments of the world when so much of it lay in ruins.

Thousands of people left the city. I lost my job. I couldn't find any form of employment. I sat in my apartment scrolling through online job boards with growing desperation. One day Miriam called me to say that a model had walked out of her still-life class complaining of the cold and would I like to come and replace him. The school paid about ten bucks an hour and all I would need to do was stand still. I biked down to the art school. I took off my clothes and stood in front of the art students while they drew sketches of my likeness.

I embraced the absurdity of my position, remembering random summer jobs I had done in England as a teenager, dressing up as a medieval king for tourists, digging trenches in the ground, walking through cornfields picking weeds, as if none of it was real, like I was some dumb character in a movie, but the sense of distance soon collapsed. The dumb character was me. In the eyes of the world, my worth had collapsed to the status of a physical object, a lump of meat to stare at and register in height and width and girth.

As the holidays approached, I saw an ad in the local paper for seasonal workers in a toy store. I was hired as a toy demonstrator. I demonstrated the nascent artificial intelligence of a robot dog called Aibo. He had six distinct poses, his manufacturer said, mimicking six recognizable human emotions. Now and then I'd demonstrate the karaoke machine. One day I was singing "Nowhere Man" by the Beatles when a customer came up to me and said, "Don't give up your day job." "But this is my day job," I said. Every day, all day, I would listen to the store jingle playing over the loudspeakers:

> Hear the clock tick-tock while the children play.
> Let the fun and laughter chase all cares away.
> It's a time for joy for all the girls and boys.
> Welcome to our world of toys.

I must have heard those words a hundred thousand times as I skated in circles around the store, feeling the clock of my life tick-tock, remembering the Oxford scholar I once had been and imagining what that guy would think about the Nowhere Man I had become. It occurred to me that thousands of people had died in the Twin Towers and that my suffering by comparison was trivial and meaningless. Years later I would learn the expression "Compare and despair": Nothing good can come from comparing your misery to someone worse off and judging your own as unworthy. Look to others in pain and understand that nobody is spared. Use that awareness to cultivate compassion and the energy you need to commit yourself to the liberation of all sentient beings. But if you break your leg, don't look at the person in the bed next to you with two broken legs and dismiss your own leg pain as undeserving. Join the brotherhood of the broken ones. Join the sisterhood of survivors. I understood this much later. But I did not know this at the time.

I was unemployed for a year. At last I found work as a grant writer for an education nonprofit based in Silicon Valley. For a couple of months I was relieved merely to be working. But my sense of relief soon morphed into an existential unmooring. I remembered my years as a television producer in England. I could have gone back to London. But Miriam was settled in her life in San Francisco. We spoke early in our courtship about starting a family. She was in her mid-thirties and could not wait for long. If I went to England, I would be on my own again. The thought was frightening and lonely. If I stayed in California, I was Nowhere Man. I felt stuck. Before I drove to work in the morning, I would write down memories of my childhood in England. It seemed important to me to understand what had happened to my family of origin before I started a family of my own. The memories were all jumbled together and full of holes. I persisted. I kept circling back to the same handful of disconnected images.

My focus drifted. My mind ran all over the place. *Where am I supposed to live? Should I stay here in California or go back to London? What should I do for work—stay in this dead-end job or quit and do something else? Am I ready to be a father? What happened when I was fifteen? Why are there so many holes? Why can't I fill them in?* I thought about staying and leaving and parenting and divorcing and all I could remember and had forgotten, and I thought about everything that might have been and could be and what once was yet now was not. On my drive to work, it seemed to me that I had always been there, inside a metal box separated from the other boxes whose drivers I couldn't see and didn't know and whose lives were alien to me. I stared out the window. The task at hand had shifted in some significant yet inexpressible way. At lunch I'd walk to a sandwich shop next to a little artificial lake, where one day I saw a giant blue-beaked bird land, and I remembered that the Romans saw birds as omens, and I wondered what this blue bird might mean.

A coworker had told me about a new way to find information on the internet. A couple of young computer geniuses had created what sounded to me like a digital version of the ancient lost Library of Alexandria, a portal to all the knowledge in the world, the conversion of all human knowledge into zeroes and ones and the storage of this code in an enormous computer network that spanned Earth. The global library in its resurrected digital form would ensure that nothing known to humanity would ever be lost again, its founders claimed, according to my coworker, insofar as I recalled what she told me.

I typed in the URL for Google and a white void filled my screen. I watched the cursor flash in and out of existence in the empty rectangle in the center of the void. I contemplated the question then foremost in my mind. *Why do I always feel so sad? But am I really sad? That's not quite the right word . . .* I typed the word *despair* in the search box. In a fraction of a second Google found millions of pages on my chosen topic. I had no idea there was so much despair in the world. I found a book called *The Philosophy of Despair*, published in 1902 by David Starr Jordan, the first president of Stanford University.[3] He was an expert on fish and a proponent of eugenics who covered up the unsolved murder by strychnine poisoning in February 1905 of Jane Stanford, cofounder of the eponymous university.

In our youth, Jordan argues, you contemplate infinite and impossible questions. You acquire more knowledge. But knowledge is futile unless it inspires action. Thus, you must act. Without action, you fall into pessimism. And the nature of that action is of the utmost significance. "The thing you do should be for you the most important thing in the world," writes Jordan. "If you could do something better than you are doing now, everything considered, why are you not doing it?"

I stared out the window at the office parking lot. *Am I doing the most important thing in the world to me right now? No.* I fled the building and drove at ninety miles an hour to the beach. I parked my car and put on my thick black neoprene suit and strode into the roiling waters with my surfboard and dropped it onto the surface of the water and paddled across the shore break. Paddle, paddle, paddle: my passage through the whitewater could sometimes take an hour. But then I was out past the break, far from shore, waiting for the swells to form on the horizon.

I seldom caught a wave. For the most part, I fell beneath them. There always came a moment when I would know that I was falling. I would see a swell loom into view. The swell would build to a near-vertical wall, towering fifteen feet above. I would swing my board to face the beach and paddle with all my might, struggling with every sinew to propel my board to match the velocity of the wave. Then I would sense the wave jack up behind me, forming a monstrous dark presence in the periphery of my vision. I would see the wave fall below me, extending from peak to trough like two flights of stairs. I would feel myself tumble through the air toward the surface of the water and crash down into the cold, dark chaos, surrendering to the knowledge that now there was nothing to be done: in an instant the wave would collapse and I would be lost and thrashed about in the darkness, the breaking wave pounding me with several tons of avalanching whitewater, as I floundered helpless in the void, powerless to do anything except submit to the larger forces then spinning me through space, a dark chaos of such violence I would lose all sense of which direction to swim for air. Yet in the end, I always knew, the wave would release me, and I would find my way to the surface and breathe again.

I must have endured a thousand such frigid ocean beatings. Every icy assault induced a transient numb amnesia for my cares. Yet upon the thawing of my body, my bad feelings returned, no less acute than in the past. In time I came to realize that my feelings demanded my attention.

They would not be ignored. I couldn't run from them or smash them into submission. I needed to understand them.

BACK AT WORK, one day I clicked through the folder architecture of my computer hard drive, searching for a folder in which I kept my personal documents. A message appeared on my screen that said: "You are at the highest level. There is no folder above this one."

There was too much I couldn't remember. So much still didn't make sense. It felt like something had happened a long time ago, something incomprehensible, like time had exploded into pieces and I couldn't put it back together. But if forward movement on the trail of life required my understanding of the dark path behind me, what then? Absent a sci-fi DeLorean, how could I understand my past and make sense of it when it had vanished without a trace?

"You need therapy," said Miriam. Back in England we would say that to poke fun at each other. *You must be bloody mental, mate—you need therapy!* I had heard about therapy on television. But in my twenty-nine years in England I had never met anyone who had gone to speak with a living, breathing psychotherapist. It sounded like the kind of measure a person would resort to only in a state of genuine desperation, when something had gone horribly wrong with them. But Miriam's comment was devoid of derision or irony. Her wish was sincere and her matter-of-fact tone conveyed the message that all Californians went to therapy and took pills when they were sad. Britons had cornflakes for breakfast; Californians sprinkled citalopram on their gluten-free granola.

I entered an office and took my seat opposite a calm man with a beard and a professorial manner. His name was Dr. Jensen. He was a psychiatrist. I looked at him, expecting him to speak. He stared at me in silence for a while and then said, "Why don't you tell me what's on your mind."

The Time It's Always Been

I could see the tree line, where I knew the trail led down through the forest all the way to Gran's house. The house was full of old things: a Maori mask from New Zealand on the wall and old leather-bound books on the shelves, like a twelve-volume edition of *One Thousand and One Nights*, and bits of driftwood Gran had picked up on the beach and decorated with shells. In the early mornings I would go to Gran's bed and pretend that the bedclothes were mountains through which my teddy bears traveled on long and wild adventures. Anything could happen in those imaginary mountains. Sometimes when my bears came home from the mountains I would lie on my front and let Gran stroke my back underneath my pajama top. The trace of her hand making circles on my skin felt calm and lovely. In the evening I would sit by the fire in my tartan dressing gown after swimming in the cold sea with Gran, or climbing in the hills up through the gorse and bracken, and then I would lie in bed while outside the rain poured down, and listen to the roar of the wind through the trees and the raindrops pelting the window and feel the bedclothes wrapped around me. I felt so safe and warm in bed at night in my grandmother's house, underneath the mountain by the sea.

The steep, winding trail started in a forest near the sea a few hundred yards from Gran's house and followed a river up to a stone wall at the saddle between two mountains, above the tree line. There, the path to the right led to the summit of a smaller mountain, while the path to the left led to the summit of Slieve Donard, the tallest mountain in Northern Ireland. From the top of Slieve Donard I could see the town and the beach and the Irish Sea. On a summer afternoon when I was about ten, it took the four of us—me, Mummy, Daddy, and my little brother, Sebastian—most of the afternoon to reach the top. Standing on the summit, I gazed at the dark green hills surrounding me in the north and south and west and at the beach almost three thousand feet below and at the gray blue sea stretching far away toward the eastern horizon.

LONG AGO THERE WAS nothing, and it was timeless and infinite. Being exploded from nothingness: space and time and matter, cosmic runaways through the emptiness, spiraling through the eons into stars and worlds and living things, and one day a naked ape stood upon the Earth, gazing at the sunrise, wondering at the light above him and how it came to be there and what it meant to him.

There were two lights, he realized. One was the light in the sky. The other was the light within him: self-awareness. *I exist*, he thinks. *I can look at the mountain on the horizon and when I close my eyes, I can see the mountain in my mind and remember my wish to go there.* His eyes open. He runs toward the mountain.

In the beginning there were no words, only sound and feeling. *Baboom baboom*: I hear the primordial rhythm of the womb. I have no conception of past or future. I am outside of time, outside the world organized into separate things like shoes and spoons that persist in time and space. I am not yet separate from the Giant One, this magic being from whence I came and whose arms and gaze form a sphere around me. There are lights and sounds and strange emanations from inside that come out as cries and giggles, and I see eyes watching over me and feel arms that circle around my little body. This moment is the universe. Leave me alone and being alone is all that I know. I have no words or thoughts but the feelings to which my mother's mind gives form. One kind of cry means *hungry*, another means *tired*. Now a need has a name attached to it.

A nascent self emerges, a rhythm of being and nothingness, embodied in the mind's emergent core, a music of light and sound and feeling. Around me there are hands and light and the gaze of the Giant One. The big hands keep me warm. I exist inside this sphere of the magic being above me and her gaze. It is a kind of dream, a space where the two minds run together. I come to feel a rhythm in the way the light becomes the darkness and turns back again to light, the way the cold and hunger form the feeling that forms the cry that summons the hands that turn the cold into the warmth and the hunger into milk.

Then I come to know another rhythm. I feel it in the way the Giant One comes and goes, when I feel her presence and when she disappears, when I am seen and when I become invisible, when fear turns into a cry that summons hands that turn the fear into calm, into the assurance that my cry can be heard. My tiny hands reach out to grasp the hands of the Giant One. Soon, I'm moving by myself, wriggling on my belly across the floor. Eyes that once watched from the outside become a sense on the inside, deep down in the parts of me that formed in the wordless flow of sound and feeling in the womb, of an invisible circle linking me to the Giant One.

Picture a woman in her early twenties. Trendy white jacket. Brown hair, beautiful, smiling, brown eyes radiant with adoration. A baby in her arms, asleep, wrapped in a yellow blanket and the feeling of being held. Mama and baby: *Mummy*, I called her. I found this picture of my mother and me in a box of photos in her flat in England when I went to see her following her fall almost half a century later. There was a handwritten document in the box that listed the times that she fed me when I was twelve days old: 2:35 a.m., 3:20, 6:45, 7:20, 9:10, 1:40 p.m., and 5:25 p.m.

My parents were both in their early twenties when I was born. My father had read *Doctor Spock's Baby and Child Care*, the parenting bible of the era. But unlike his Vulcan namesake, Spock the childcare guru didn't know everything. My parents were on their own, a young couple from Ireland, a Protestant man and Catholic woman at the peak of Ireland's centuries-long sectarian war, migrating to a safer life in England, someplace where they could be together and build a home, doing their best to take care of a baby. "It's like children having children," said a Belfast college friend of my father, poking fun at him.

I am told that my first word other than *Daddy* and *Mummy* was *carry*. "Mummy carry," I said. "You said that anytime you were upset," my father told me. *Mummy carry*: sometimes I can still feel the hole where her arms used to be.

In the middle of the rolling green hills of southern England stands a vast and ancient cathedral. History doesn't record the image that once appeared on its stained-glass window. Perhaps it showed the faces of God and the Holy Family. Nobody will ever know. Long ago someone smashed the window into pieces. Legend blames a soldier in the English Civil War who launched a cannon attack at the cathedral from a nearby hill. One of the soldier's cannonballs soared from the hill and went through the window. The faces became a pile of shattered fragments on the ground. The people of the town tried to put the window back together. They remembered the beauty of the original faces and yearned to see them again. But the task of solving this giant jigsaw puzzle proved impossible. The new window showed none of the old faces, just a kaleidoscope of broken pieces, reassembled in an abstract form. It fit the space but would never match the original. The area where the soldier staged his attack was known centuries later as Cannon Road. By the early 1970s it was a peaceful, leafy neighborhood on the edge of a quiet town of thirty thousand souls. When I was four, my parents bought a house there.

Later, memories of my boyhood years were likewise shattered into a thousand broken pieces. I have put the fragments of my childhood memory back together in my mind. I was always waiting for something. Waiting for the weekend. Waiting for my birthday or Easter Sunday or Christmas Day. Waiting for *Doctor Who* on Saturday night television. Waiting for the bell to ring or sweets after supper, waiting for the referee to blow the whistle, so I could get out of the freezing rain and go home with numb hands and feet and lie in my hot bath and feel the chilblains aching in all my limbs but then taste the creamy deliciousness of the cocoa that Mummy brought up to the bathtub. Waiting for the start of summer, for the morning when the chestnut trees were sprouting again, all bushy and green, rustling in the breeze with their flowery cones, little branches dancing against my window, saying, *Hello, hello, wake up*, and I would hear the birds again saying, *Coo-coo, coo-coo*, and on the way to school, someone would say, "Race ya!" and all the boys would take off, sprinting toward the trees, and for a while I would be neck and neck with the others, but then I would feel my legs speed up and I would surge to the front and sense the other boys falling far behind me, as I ran faster and even faster, until I could see nothing else in front of me except the empty field.

I liked being fast. I liked being first. It meant the teachers would see me. They would tell me I was good and clever. They would tell me I knew the right answer. I liked that. I liked knowing things. I would sit at the front of the class with my hand stretched high in the air, begging my teacher to call on me. Her name was Mrs. Mahon. I would give her my answer, and she would tell me I was right, and I would feel so good inside, because I knew things. I knew that the speed of light was 186,282 miles per second. I knew that plants and animals were made of cells and that inside the cells of animals was DNA, which stood for deoxyribonucleic acid. And I knew that inside my head was my brain and that the brain was what told my body what to do. I knew so many things.

I understood that there were limits to my knowledge. Looking south from the summit of Donard, a few miles over the horizon, I could see the little fishing town where Mummy grew up with Granny. Granny was Mummy's mummy. But not her real mummy. Her real mummy was a model. Her real daddy was a soldier from the US who was sent to Ireland with the army to fight the German soldiers on the beaches in Normandy. After World War II the model and the soldier gave Mummy away to a priest when she was eighteen months old, then ran away without her to America. The priest gave Mummy to Granny and Grandpa. Granny had grown up with her ten sisters and brothers on a farm and had dentures because one day when she was little a goat kicked her in the face and smashed all the teeth from her mouth.

Grandpa was a laborer who had returned from England, where he had helped build the first motorway in Britain. Granny and Grandpa couldn't have a baby, so the priest gave them Mummy, but Mummy didn't know about her real parents until she was ten and one of the girls at school said, "Clara, you're *adapted*," because that was how the word *adopted* sounded with a Northern Ireland accent, only Mummy didn't know the word or what the girl was talking about, and she wondered what it meant to be adapted, and from the sound of the girl's teasing voice it sounded like being adapted was bad. When she ran home from school, she told Granny about the girl, and Granny told her about the model and the soldier, and Granny said the soldier was a big man who came to the house once, but that was all she said and all she knew, and she was sorry she never told wee Clara before, but she had been scared that Clara would run away if she ever found out she wasn't really Granny's natural child, and that sure would be dreadful, would it not, because Granny loved wee Clara and that was why she got her that smart uniform and sent her to the school, where Clara learned to sing and got medals for Irish dancing, and yes, there was the time when she was little and playing by a Primus stove and it fell on her and she caught on fire and still had that brown patch on her face that looked like freckles, but that had been an accident, and sure, she didn't pass the exam for grammar school, so she went to the nuns who gave her those bad dreams, but they taught her to read and write so she could go to technical school and learn to type so she got a job as a typist and met that lovely Protestant fella with the long beard, home from college in Belfast, though it was an awful shame, sure it was, that some of his family hated Catholics because of all the bombs and killings, so when they got married they had to run away from Ireland.

I knew that sometimes I had to run away as well. One time, on the way down Slieve Donard, Daddy said, "Why don't you run on ahead"—although maybe it was Mummy, or Daddy echoing her wishes, or my impression of their wishes combined in a single presence. I can't remember what happened before I heard those words. I can remember thinking something like *Well, all right then. I'll show you.* I must have felt belittled or angry. I set off running down the mountain. I was amazed how fast I flew downhill. I let my legs spin round, and gravity pulled me in a matter of minutes down a trail that had taken us hours to ascend. I sped downhill, jumping left and right over little piles of loose granite fragments, feeling such joy in the experience of becoming as close to airborne as an animal without wings could hope for, how the mere intention of pointing myself downhill and allowing gravity to take hold aligned my body with the full downward force of Earth. As the path through the tree line came into view, an idea took shape in my mind.

Run on ahead: I understood there was a limit to how far *ahead* meant I was supposed to go. When we went on walks in the woods near our house in England, *ahead* meant round the next corner, or the corner after that at most. But it wasn't an exact distance, like a meter or a light-year. So the instruction had given me a sort of freedom. That was good, because now I had the dark, angry feeling that Mummy and Daddy called *sulking*. You could tell me I was the worst little boy on Earth and it wouldn't matter, because I was done listening. Done. You could tell me I shouldn't keep making that sulky face because the wind might change and my face would get stuck like that forever, and I'd think, *Okay, good. I like my sulky face, and I like the thought of you having to look at me looking back at you and knowing I won't stop sulking—never, never, never, not until the sun blows up and swallows Earth and all the stars flicker out and die.* So the dark feeling was good because now I could run on ahead. I could run to Gran's house.

But I didn't like the dark feeling. It meant I was bad. I was supposed to be a Good Boy. And how hard I tried to be good! I cleaned my teeth and said my prayers. I knew my twelve times table. I got two gold stars from Mrs. Mahon for my horror story about the killer on the run from the police. I read so many books that on parents' night Mrs. Mahon said I had "swallowed the encyclopedia," and as well as the first two pages of Jayant Narlikar's *The Structure of the Universe*, I could even read the long, hard books that Mummy was reading for her degree. Early in the morning before school I would see her downstairs by the electric fire, bundled in a wooly sweater with her cup of steaming coffee and her notebook and all her squiggly writing in it and the big stack of thick books in front of her. She had gone back to school. She didn't want to be a typist anymore. She wanted to be a teacher. "Sit down," she said one day, and opened one of the books. She showed me a page with lots of big words. "*Prelapsarian*—it means before the Fall," she said. "But not like the actual Fall, when Adam and Eve left the Garden of Eden. It's a metaphor. Do you understand?" "Yes, Mummy," I said. I did. Then she told me she had received some wisdom from one of her professors in response to a paper she had written that she wanted to pass on to me. "Remember that you must always use words in the right way," she said. "You can't make words mean *whatever you like*." "All right, Mummy," I said.

Always use words in the right way. It was as if Mummy was Alice and I was Humpty Dumpty, in the bit in *Through the Looking-Glass* by Lewis Carroll when Humpty Dumpty tells Alice words mean whatever he chooses them to mean, because in the end all that matters, according to Humpty Dumpty, is who is the master of them. But I knew what Alice knew and a long word like *prelapsarian* and what a metaphor was and how there were different meanings of *Fall*, and I knew that knowing this was the clever part of me, which meant that I was good.

But I also knew about the bad part inside me. I was a sinner. When Adam ate from the Tree of the Knowledge of Good and Evil, he got free will, but God threw him and Eve out of Eden because they had broken the rules of the original garden. There was the time I didn't take my books back to the library and got so worried about what would happen if Mummy found out, I took the books to a field and buried them. There was the time I told Sebastian to close his eyes and open his mouth and I shoved in a fistful of sand. There was the time I built a platform out of Legos at the top of the stairs and told him to sit down on it. "No," he said, "you'll push me off." "I promise I won't," I said. Sebastian sat down. I shoved him as hard as I could. His skinny body soared into the air and collapsed on the floor with a thud. Daddy heard the thud and Sebastian crying and came running. "Father Christmas won't be coming this year," Daddy said. Then he made us hold hands and sing the song we sang after fighting. *"Make friends, make friends, never, never break friends. Because if you do, you'll catch the flu, and that will be the end of you."*

Then there was the time I hid sweets in my boots. When Mummy was in the kitchen, she would send me to pick up milk or margarine at the local shop. I would buy the milk or margarine with the pound note Mummy had given me, then visit the bakery across the street and buy myself a little cake and scoff the whole thing leaning against a tree in the woods. It felt so good, sitting there in the sunshine, eating something yummy. I knew it was bad. A good Catholic boy like me was never supposed to steal. Mummy said so. Mrs. Mahon said so. Father Tim and the Bible said so. Good boys went to heaven. Bad boys went to hell. But what was one little cake to Jesus? He would surely forgive me. And besides, Mummy never noticed. I would finish the cake and walk home and give Mummy the milk or margarine and the change from her pound note and then go back for more cake the next time.

One day she counted the change and asked me why milk cost so much. "Inflation," I said. She nodded. *But wouldn't it be so nice*, I thought sometime later, *if instead of needing to scoff the cake in the woods, I could take a little something home and eat it watching television.* I devised a plan. It was sunny outside when I walked to the shop, conspicuous on a dry and cloudless lunchtime in my black rubber Wellington boots. I went to the candy section. I looked at the Revels and Space Dust and Mars and Maltesers and Bounty and Twix and Marathon, and the thought of all the wondrous sensations in store for me when I smuggled them back home and crept upstairs and went into my room and lay down on my bed and turned on my little black-and-white television and watched *The Six Million Dollar Man* sucking each morsel of chocolate one at a time until they dissolved in my saliva filled me with the joy of giving myself an early Christmas and Easter all rolled into one. How I loved chocolate! At Christmas and Easter, I was allowed to eat as much as I wanted. On Christmas morning I would eat six candy bars before the sun was up. The rest of the year, the rule was three sweets after lunch and supper, except on Saturdays, when I was allowed a Zoom lollipop along with my *Buster* comic.

I put the candy packets in my pockets. The candy made the pockets stick out, so I put the candy in my boots. I went home. As I walked through the front door into the kitchen, the candy made a crunching sound. Step, crunch, step, crunch. I put the milk on the counter. I handed the margarine and change to Mummy and turned to go upstairs. "What's inside your boots?" she said.

"Nothing," I said. "I don't believe you," she said. "Take off your boots." I took them off. The candy tumbled onto the floor. "Go to your room," she said. I went upstairs and lay on the bed and burst into sobs.

An eternity passed. *I'm bad. Evil. A liar and a glutton and a thief.* I cried until my eyes stopped making tears and then I kept on crying. More time passed. *I deserve to be here as long as Mummy wants me to.* The lonely torture of abandonment coursed through every cell in my little mind and body, until at last my mother decided my punishment had ended and responded to my cry. "Are you crying because you're sorry," she said, entering the room, "or because I found you out?" It was like a riddle. I didn't know what to say. "Because I'm sorry," I said. She nodded and left the room.

And then there was the time I was so bad Mummy turned into a ghost. One night I was in the bathtub with Sebastian when I had an idea to play a trick on Mummy. "I'll go underwater and close my eyes and hold my breath and make myself lie still," I said. "Then when Mummy comes in and asks you what happened, you tell her that I'm dead." "Okay," said Sebastian. Mummy came into the bathroom. She saw me lying totally still underwater. I heard Sebastian say the words

I had told him to say. The next thing I knew, Mummy was picking me up out of the tub and holding me under one arm and dragging me out of the bathroom and down the hall toward the top of the stairs. "Mummy, I'm okay!" I said. But she didn't hear me. Didn't even notice I was there. This horrid feeling came over me like I was stuck inside a bad dream but couldn't wake up. I tried to wriggle out of Mummy's grasp. She held on tight. I could see she had this weird frozen look on her face. She kept repeating Daddy's name in this low, scary ghost voice: "Joseph . . . Joseph . . . Joseph . . ." I saw Mummy again just before I went to bed. She was sitting by herself in the dining room. She had her head in her hands. I went up next to her. "Sorry," I said. She was silent. I went upstairs. I knelt by my bed. I said three Our Fathers and two Hail Marys and I told Jesus I was sorry for being bad. "I promise to be a good boy," I said. "I'll never be bad again."

I knew that something weird had happened the night when Mummy turned into a ghost. It felt like she disappeared. Or I disappeared. Or both of us. She was always disappearing. I didn't know why. I didn't like to think about it. Once when I was very little I was sitting in our van. I was looking through the window at the row of houses. Mummy had gone into one of them. I didn't know why. I waited and waited and waited, and I needed to go number two, but still there was no sign of her, and I didn't know what I was supposed to do, and I cried and yelled until I couldn't hold it anymore. Then Mummy came back and drove home and took me upstairs, and I stood in the tub while she washed all the poo off my legs.

Another time I was alone in the house, staring through the upstairs window at the dark, empty driveway. *Where did they go? They've been gone for ages and ages.* I looked outside at the oak tree and the dark hedges. I went downstairs to the living room. I went back to the top of the stairs to look outside again. *What if they're dead?* The horrid feeling came. I didn't know what to do. I went back downstairs to the living room and turned on the television. I tried to watch some old black-and-white film that was on. All I could think about was how Mummy and Daddy and Sebastian might be dead. I stared at the screen as long as I could stand it. *When I go back and look at the driveway, I will see them.* I looked at the screen. I waited some more. I went back to the window. Nothing. *They must be dead.* My heart beat faster and faster. I ran out the front door onto the driveway. I stared into the darkness down the road. I ran to our neighbors' house. I knocked on the door. The nice old lady who lived there opened the door. Her name was Mrs. John. She lived in the house with her husband and their big brown dog Megan. If I kicked a ball by accident into their garden, Mrs. John didn't mind if I climbed the fence to go and get the ball. "Mummy and Daddy and Sebastian went to town a long time ago," I said. "I don't know where they are!" Mrs. John told me to come inside. "Why don't you play with Megan," she said. I stroked the dog until the horrible feeling went away and I heard the crunch of car wheels on the gravel of our driveway and knew that Mummy and Daddy and Sebastian were still alive.

One day the future went dark. It is hard to pin down when looking forward turned from delight to terror, when the future became a dreadful vision I devoted almost all my conscious effort to shield myself from seeing. Perhaps the darkness started when I saw the boy with the burns. Once I knew of his existence, it was impossible to imagine what it might have felt like not to know about him. I kept on seeing him. I had to. I did not know why. It happened every time I found myself browsing through the bookshelves in the living room. Our house was full of books. Books in the kitchen. Books in the playroom and bedrooms, and thousands in the living room. Books on astronomy and birds and cooking and religion. Sci-fi novels, poetry, old hardbacks that Daddy had inherited from ancestors in Ireland, like *Atlantis: The Book of the Angels*, the autobiography of an archangel who had witnessed the destruction of the legendary lost continent, transcribed by a Victorian author called D. Bridgman-Metchim. I loved to look at its monochrome illustrations. The first image, facing the title page, depicted a thin humanlike figure leaping across a moonlit sky. I could look at the pictures in *Atlantis* for a long time, and then I might read the first few pages of *The Structure of the Universe*, the parts before the book filled with big words and weird symbols I didn't understand. Then I would watch my hand reach down to the lower shelf with Daddy's books from his volunteer work for the Campaign for Nuclear Disarmament, and I would pick up the Hiroshima book again.

I opened the book. I saw the mushroom cloud, the gray and black and monstrous entity rising from the city. I saw the ruined buildings and the shadows of human beings left on the broken walls. My heart beat faster, and a horrid feeling washed over me and into me. I turned the page. There was the boy. He lay on a hospital bed. Against the pure white sheets, his bare legs were charcoal black with nuclear flash burns. How such a horrible thing had come into the world was beyond all reason. And yet it existed. It was a nightmare transcending the evilest imagination. But I knew the boy was not imaginary. A quarter-century before I was born, the Americans dropped an atom bomb on Hiroshima. Little Boy, they called it. All the houses blew into pieces, and the people turned into ash and vapor. The book did not state what had happened to the boy. Maybe he was dead now. Maybe alive. I wished that I knew if he was dead or living. I wished that he really was just a figment of someone's dark imagination. Then I could go back to the life I had had before I saw him, looking forward to Christmas and Easter and the summer and the autumn and then another Christmas again, around and around in the endless wheel of time.

But there was no going back. Once you knew something, there was no unknowing it. The atomic bomb was real. The boy was real. And now more bombs were on the horizon. American missiles were coming to England in 1983. Three years. I would be twelve then. Three summers, three birthdays, three Christmases and Easters. Then the nuclear war would happen. The thought was too large and frightening to fit inside my head. But it was true. Daddy said so. So it had to be true. He knew things. One time at Gran's house in Ireland I found his school report book. One of his teachers had said he was "in a class of his own." He went to college when he was sixteen and got a first in mathematics and astronomy and worked as a computer programmer, in the era when computers were the size of refrigerators and nobody had one at home. I felt like he could fly to the moon. With his shoulder-length curly hair and long hippie beard, he looked like the pictures of Jesus I saw on the Stations of the Cross in church. Imagine a computer genius Jesus telling you something was true: I trusted him.

At the weekend we would go on marches to the US Air Force base, 30 miles away. Light traveled at 186,282 miles per second. If the Americans put missiles on the base and had a nuclear war with Russia, it was no good being only 30 miles away. Everyone would die. Me, Mummy, Daddy, Sebastian, Briar, all my friends and teachers, Mrs. John and Megan: all dead. I marched with a sign I'd made out of a breakfast cereal box. I drew a mushroom cloud with my colored pencils. My sign said: I WANT TO GROW UP NOT BLOW UP. Sometimes I would listen to a song in Daddy's record collection called "Enola Gay" by OMD. That was the name of the bomber that had dropped Little Boy on Hiroshima at eight fifteen one August morning thirty-five years earlier: *Enola Gay*. *"It's eight fifteen, and that's the time it's always been,"* went the song. The nuclear missiles were coming to the base in three years, Daddy said. People used to say that World War III was "unthinkable." The US and Russia had so many nuclear bombs, the war would kill everyone in the world. All the dust from all the bombs might even block out the sun for centuries, killing all the plants and animals too.

But now a third world war was thinkable. Some insane generals had a mad plan. Russia had put nuclear missiles in Eastern Europe. The US would put them in England. Then the US and Russia would have a nuclear war in Europe, while they stayed safe on the sidelines. It seemed unfair that children like me had to suffer in the middle of this grown-up madness. It wasn't my fault that the US and Russia hated each other, but their hatred was going to kill me. I had three years until the missiles came. Three years until the end of the world. *I'll be twelve—that's three more birthdays and Christmases. I hope it's over quick.*

I could go for days and forget all about the third world war. But then

I'd be walking down the road to school and remember. The knowledge would flash back into my head like an H-bomb of the mind. My heart would beat faster. All the trees and the sky and the ground would feel dreamlike and unreal. I could see everything burning white and the mushroom cloud coming out of the ground. I felt the world was ending in that very moment. *Don't think about it*, I would tell myself. If I waited long enough, the fear would go away, and I would forget again about this horrible thing I knew but didn't want to know. How other people handled knowing it, I had no idea. Sometimes I would watch the other boys and girls on the playing field at school, laughing and running about, and marvel at the minds so strong that they could shield themselves from the awful feeling or even from the knowledge itself.

One night I woke from a nightmare, feeling such a weight of dread and panic that I realized I could not hope to lie there alone and wait for the feeling to pass. I went downstairs. My father was watching television. "Daddy, what will happen if we can't stop the missiles?" I said. I had no idea what I wanted him to say. I wanted to believe that the mad generals were not the only power in the world, that the rest of us, the ordinary people who just wanted to live our lives, would prevail. Then I could go to bed, knowing I was safe. But what Daddy said was "I don't know," so I went back to my room and closed my eyes and prayed to God, asking him to please stop the nuclear missiles coming to England and to please protect me and Sebastian and Mummy and Daddy and all the people in the world from the third world war, and I tried not to imagine all the world on fire, all the mushroom clouds in London and New York and Los Angeles and Moscow and Berlin and Paris and all the children in every city of the world stumbling about the ruins with their stunned, sad faces and their burnt skin sloughing off their bodies like rags.

YOU CAN'T FEAR THE past, only the future. The past can't hurt you. It already happened. But fear can play funny tricks on the mind. "Fear of breakdown is the fear of a breakdown that has already been experienced," wrote the twentieth-century British pediatrician and psychoanalyst D. W. Winnicott.[4] My nuclear fears seemed to be about an apocalyptic future. I wasn't delusional: threats of nuclear conflict did loom on the geopolitical horizon. But looking back, I can see how the level of isolation and panic I experienced had an exaggerated quality, even within the context of objective danger. It strikes me in hindsight that what I was afraid of wasn't entirely in the future. I was afraid of some kind of explosion that had already started happening. Perhaps it was easier to imagine that the danger—however horrific—was on the outside, in the Pentagon and the Kremlin and Greenham Common, separated in space and time from the solid world of my home. Perhaps the really unbearable thought would have been to sense the collapse of the solid world of home, even perhaps to wonder if it had ever truly been solid, to worry that there was a dark and frightening state of being not on the outside but invading the present moment, a world without a mother to carry me.

And so when I later would recall the day on the mountain and the dark feeling that sent me running, it was hard not to think of the boy with the burns and sometimes even imagine that wounded boy running down the mountain along with me.

I'll show you what running ahead looks like, I thought. I sped down the mountain, down the path that led into the trees. I knew the path led the whole way down the mountain and to the seaside house where Gran lived. *I'll run to Gran's house. How amazing that will be! Mummy and Daddy will be so proud of me. Their son just ten years old, and he ran down a mountain!* I followed the path. I wound through the trees and came to the street where Gran lived. I knocked on the door. She wasn't home. I sat on the chair outside the door and waited. Time passed. I didn't understand what might be taking them so long. Then I saw Daddy marching down the street. His face was bright red like a tomato. His forehead was covered with sweat. "Daddy, I'm here!" I said. He was angry. "Where the bloody hell have you been?" he said. Something had gone wrong that day, and I didn't know why. But I knew that I had done something amazing. I had run down a mountain, and forever after, whenever the dark feeling came, I knew I could fly through the air as close to airborne as any wingless creature, feeling the cycle of earth becoming air, the terrestrial and the heavenly, feeling the ground beneath my feet with every step, and hearing Earth say, *I am here.*

Ball, Book, Flag

I finished my speech for Dr. Jensen, imagining he might give me a medal for a stunning level of insight displayed by a first-time patient, but instead he said, "While you've obviously done a great deal of thinking about your past, I wonder how much consideration you might have given as to why it could be difficult for you to let it go."

Let go of *what*? What happened when I ran down the mountain? How it felt to find the sleeping hedgehog in the Jungle? The feeling of Gran's hand on my back, and the smell of the autumn leaves in the garden? Drop all my precious jewels of childhood memory in the trash can of personal history—was that my psychiatrist's professional opinion? I wasn't sure I was willing. And let's say I was. How did a person accomplish such a thing? By talking about it? Really? How was talking about memories I couldn't let go meant to accomplish anything except make them even more memorable?

MERCURY WAS THE MESSENGER between mortal humans and the gods. The Romans called him Hermes. Hermes flew back and forth between Earth and Mount Olympus, carrying messages. Nineteenth-century scholars of the humanities likened the sources of human knowledge to Mount Olympus and the interpretation of those sources to Hermes. The word *hermeneutics*, the philosophy of interpretation, is a coinage in tribute to Hermes. To understand the whole meaning of a book or historical period, you need to examine its component parts. Know more about the parts, and you expand your perception of the whole. Know more about the whole, and you see the parts in a new light. This cycle from whole to part and back again—what the twentieth-century German philosopher Martin Heidegger called the *hermeneutic circle*—constitutes the process of historical understanding: the loops of remembering and reinterpreting through which we understand the meaning of the past, whether collective or personal. There is a hermeneutics of everything, from the meaning of scripture to the history of America, from the significance of ancient myth to the story of your life. Your mind travels back to the old days. Time passes. When your thoughts return to the old days again, you see the past from a different perspective, yielding knowledge that in turn transforms your experience of the present moment, like a series of messages conveyed by Mercury from Mount Olympus.

Nothing is permanent. Loss is inevitable. Memory is how we preserve knowledge from loss. Nowadays we outsource memory to the internet. But it used to be an art form. The ancients understood memory as humanity's principal defense against the inexorable ravages of time. An understanding of memory's interrelationship with tragedy is implicit in a pioneering memorization technique, devised in ancient Rome, known as the memory palace. Cicero described the origin of memory palaces in *De Oratore*: The poet Simonides attended a dinner in a banquet hall. The building collapsed. Simonides ran out of the building and survived. Later he managed to remember the names of the people crushed in the ruins by visualizing their positions around the banquet table. You can remember anything using the technique Simonides discovered, said Cicero. Visualize a building. Imagine yourself walking through the building. For every item you want to remember, substitute a vivid image and place it in one of the imaginary rooms.

Centuries later the Renaissance astronomer and alchemist Giordano Bruno rediscovered the Roman memory method and elaborated on it with a complex mnemonic system. Inspired by Hermetic texts from the first century CE, Bruno linked the secret virtues of stones and plants with the power of the stars, reflecting the alchemical vision of a cosmic symmetry between microcosm and macrocosm—the universe in a grain of sand. In the famous words of a Hermetic text called *The Emerald Tablet*: "As above, so below."

Bruno first outlined his approach in a late sixteenth-century text entitled *De Umbris Idearum* (*On the Shadows of Ideas*). "Shadow is not darkness," wrote Bruno, "but rather shadow is the tracing of trails in light, or the sign of light in darkness." In the back of his book, Bruno drew a circle. "Move around this circle in your mind," said Bruno. "Contemplate the entire contents of your mind and the links between the world below and the world above, the inner and the outer, and you will comprehend all things and know the meaning that binds the All in the One: the secret knowledge in the shadows."[5]

Bruno's obscure magical memory systems faded into historical oblivion. In the era following Bruno's execution by the Catholic Church, for his dabbling in the occult and his heretical belief that the universe contains an infinite number of stars, the alchemical art of memory was superseded by the scientific understanding of the mind. The pioneering neurologists and psychiatrists of the nineteenth century, like Pierre Janet and Sigmund Freud, were interested in a different sort of shadow: the enduring effects on the body and mind of psychological trauma. Where Bruno directed his reader to rotate imaginary concentric wheels, Sigmund Freud invited his patient to let their thoughts run free, talk about anything that came to their mind, and, in so doing, illuminate the links between the surface level of their conscious awareness—the nightmares, paralysis, and other baffling symptoms that had brought them to treatment—and the suppressed or repressed memories of terrifying experiences of assault or grief hidden in the shadow realm outside the frontier of everyday awareness: the unconscious.

The ensuing era of modern psychology and neuroscience then yielded an understanding of this shadow realm of unconscious traumatic memory in scientific terms. Most of us go around thinking of ourselves as a single, unitary entity. The self feels continuous through space and time. But this sensation of unity is an illusion, a sort of conjuring trick of evolution.

The self in reality is a constellation of states that evolve through time and vary across mood and situation. The movement from one state of mind to another is called dissociation. As the psychoanalyst Philip Bromberg wrote: "Self-states are what the mind comprises. Dissociation is what the mind does. The relationship between self-states and dissociation is what the mind is. It is the stability of that relationship that enables a person to experience continuity as 'I.'"[6]

Dissociation is a normal and healthy capacity of the mind. It is like an edit in a movie, a way of shifting from one scene of experience to the next. Under ordinary circumstances, there is nothing wrong with it. Daydreaming is a form of dissociation. To focus on anything at all, you need to collapse the circle of attention to one part of experience and split off everything else. If you're splitting off meaningless distractions, that's a useful thing to be able to do. You'll never need to remember them anyway. But when the mind splits off experiences because they're too frightening or incomprehensible to tolerate—a phenomenon known as traumatic dissociation—the feelings of horror, fear, or shame associated with the experience never fade away. Recent research on the neurophysiology of traumatic dissociation suggests that overwhelming stress releases pain-reducing chemicals that disconnect the neural networks lower in the brain that process emotion from the higher networks in the frontal cortex that support our capacity for self-awareness, reason, and memory.[7] Trauma memories linger in the shadows of consciousness, forming an atmosphere around every single moment of experience, like runaways of the mind.

Disaster strikes. Earth keeps turning around the sun. But trauma traps the mind in time, circling a nucleus of dissociated experience, like a planet in orbit around a dying star.

I COULDN'T SLEEP. I couldn't remember a single moment in my life when I hadn't felt afraid. I had always managed to keep the fear at bay. To keep moving and run ahead of the darkness. But now the darkness was catching up with me. The mysteries of my past were vexing in themselves. But the past was only one of three problems. My other two problems were the present and the future. The present was a problem because I hated my current job as a grant writer but couldn't think of what else I might want to do. Or rather, I thought of a new occupation every fifteen minutes but kept changing my mind. The future was a problem because I imagined it as a replica of the present, only worse. The future loomed like a windowless room from which no exit would ever be possible. Miriam and I had begun to speak of having children. Coming home from my long day marooned in an office cubicle, I tried to picture myself as a father—a much wiser and more calm future version of myself, a grown-up who understood his past and present and his forward path through life: it felt like science fiction. I was thirty-three years old. I had been pondering the mysteries of my childhood since I woke up one morning sad and lonely and grief-stricken seven years earlier and decided I had to know why. On that cold, dark English winter morning, I had forced myself out of bed and sat by my laptop, writing down memories of Cannon Road. For a while I could see the garden again. I could see the apple trees and the greenhouse and the leaves in the autumn, blanketing the grass, and Sebastian and I raking the leaves into piles and piling them in the wheelbarrow and pushing the barrow to the compost heap at the edge of the Jungle. For a long time, my mind circled between my cold, dark basement flat in London and this garden in memory, like Mercury circling back and forth for ages from Earth to Mount Olympus, but without ever delivering me a message I could really understand.

But after seven years of mental circling, my past remained a mystery. My anxiety intensified. I was anxious when I woke in the morning. I was anxious on my drive south on the freeway to work and in the evening driving home, contemplating the identical day that soon would follow. I became less anxious after drinking gin or wine or beer and eating ice cream and then lying down in bed, stupefied by booze and worn out by a day of worrying, but then I usually felt sad. I returned to Dr. Jensen every week for several months. He indulged my circular monologues with minimal interruption. I felt worse and worse. I begged the doctor for medicine to alleviate my suffering. He scribbled a note on his prescription pad and gave it to me. I went to the pharmacy and picked up a bottle of Klonopin. I went to a café. I sat down with a newspaper and a double latte. I opened the bottle and took out a little pink pill. I washed down the pill with a swig of foamy coffee.

A feeling of serenity washed through me. I put down the newspaper and stared out the window. *There is nothing to worry about. Nothing I need to do. I can just sit like this forever. I can let it go.* My serenity persisted for about an hour and then my anxiety returned.

I would wake in the wee hours, my heart racing, overwhelmed with terror. "I used to feel like I was going somewhere. What happened to my life? Who am I?" Miriam would hold me, saying, "Hush, darling. You're here with me now. Everything's going to be fine. I promise." Her words pacified me only for a moment. "But I don't know who I am!" I began to writhe on the bed. I wound myself into a fetal position. "Breathe, honey, breathe," said Miriam. "I can't go in there," I sobbed, meaning the office, and she said, "Well, don't go in—just call in sick," and I said, "But I have to go in!" and she said, "Well, why don't you go in for a few hours and do your best so at least you'll get something done," and then I cried, "But I can't go into that place!" and so it went on, back and forth, until I fell asleep in her arms.

In the morning, golden sunshine streamed through our apartment window curtains, consuming me with dread at the prospect of another day to get through. This sequence repeated itself night after night for months on end as I struggled with a chronic sense of panic and encroaching disaster. As each day dawned, I'd burst into tears and hold on to Miriam as if outside her arms I'd plunge through a hole into the center of the Earth.

I compiled a list of instructions for myself. I hoped the list would console my panicked self with messages from its occasionally calmer counterpart. It began as follows: "You wrote this when you were calm and rational—a sane human being! If you lose your shit, read and know the following." I then listed these instructions:

1. If you wake up in the middle of the night freaking out, get out of bed immediately! Go to the beach and get in the water. DO NOT STAY IN BED!

2. If you hear negative or self-critical thoughts, DO NOT BELIEVE THEM! SOMEONE ELSE IS TALKING!

3. Remember that Miriam loves you.

4. Remember that you love Miriam.

5. Remember that Dad and Sebastian love you.

6. If you find yourself weeping, worried, and hysterical, tell yourself, *You are a good person! You deserve to be happy!*

7. If you find yourself at work thinking, *I should never have left London . . . I should have figured out what happened in 1986 . . . I should be doing something else for work* . . . remember you can and will achieve these things in the future, but right now you need to focus! Do your work right now! Do it well!

8. You create your own experience.

9. You are doing this to yourself. You can stop it.

10. All of this will pass. Nothing is permanent.

When I awoke in a state of terror some nights later, I forgot to read my instructions, and wouldn't have believed them even if I had. I endured the following six months in a downward slide toward a chasm of despair and panic that reduced my existence to the challenge of getting through each day without bursting into tears. It was hard to know which was worse, the sadness or the terror. The sadness was a constant. It lurked in the background, underneath the fear, moving into the foreground of awareness when I went to bed at night, and in the lulls between the waves of fear. The fear came along with the inchoate perception that something was going very badly wrong. *I have to leave. RIGHT NOW. Quit my job. Go back to England. No. Then Miriam will leave me. Stay here. Look at the computer screen. Start typing again. Write the grant. "We respectfully request that the Blah Blah Foundation blah, blah, blah . . ." Oh my God, this is boring and pointless. I used to be someone. Now what am I?*

A chump in an office cubicle. This is my life now. Get out. Run. No. Stay. Runstayrunstayrunstay . . .

Insomnia and panic wore me down. The horizon of my sense of time shrunk from getting through the day to surviving the next five minutes. I started to lose my mind. My attention was the first function to go. My thoughts ran around in circles that led nowhere. Memory was next to go. I was aware of losing the ability to retain any information. It scared me. Whenever I took the train to work, I would try to memorize *Kubla Khan* by Samuel Taylor Coleridge. By the time my train reached its destination thirty minutes away, I had learned the poem by heart. But by the evening, all I could remember was Xanadu. The rest of *Kubla Khan* had vanished from my consciousness. I felt terrified.

Nothing is permanent, I had instructed myself to remember. It was true. My fear began to fade away. But in its wake came something much worse and weirder. Imagine an alien planet where it never got cold. The aliens have never encountered ice, only water. But you live on an ice world. One day the aliens communicate with you through some kind of telepathy. *Tell us about ice,* they say. *It sounds a lot like our water. It's made of the same stuff, right? Yes,* you would say. *But it has lost its ability to move. It is water in a solid state of matter. Spend too long in the frost and you go numb and freeze to death. Ice is nothing like your water. Nothing like water at all.*

I couldn't laugh. I couldn't read or write. It was even hard to speak. The problem wasn't in my tongue or vocal cords but in the parts of the mind that put experience into language. A horrifying silent chasm occupied the space where thoughts had once existed. One small mercy was my discovery that despite my loss of speech I had retained the ability to sing. I would stand at the back in the bass section of a gospel choir I had joined in a San Francisco church called Glide Memorial, and when I opened my mouth and heard the deep sound that bellowed from within me and merged with all the voices around me, the chasm inside me filled with music. One song went as follows:

I almost let go
I felt like I couldn't take life anymore
My problems had me bound
Depression weighed me down
But God held me close
So I wouldn't let go
God's mercy kept me
So I wouldn't let go
I almost gave up
I was right at the edge of a breakthrough
But I couldn't see it

When the music stopped, the silence inside me felt more terrifying than ever. I was right at the edge of a breakdown: I could feel it.

I tried other medications. I saw Dr. Jensen every week for a year and spoke without interruption for the fifty minutes of each session about the holes in my memory and the impossibility of moving forward into the future until I had understood the past. I prayed. I visited a somatic psychotherapist—someone who understood the link between the body and the mind. Ned had gone to see her. "She's different," he said. "You won't just drone on about how terrible you're feeling with the therapist just listening and never saying or doing anything." She had a soft voice and held me in her gentle gaze. She beckoned me to an armchair. She sat in a chair parallel to mine. I could sense an atmosphere of warmth between us. "Close your eyes," she said. I felt calm and safe with her. "Would it be okay if I put my hand on your forearm?" she said. "Yes," I said. I could feel the gentle touch of her hand upon my arm. I started crying. "Now I want you to try something," she said. "Would that be okay?" "Yes," I said, through tears. "Imagine somewhere that feels safe to you. Perhaps you're sitting there, perhaps moving. Picture this place where you are absolutely safe and free." I saw a trail through a forest. "Tell me what you're seeing," she said. "I'm running through the forest," I said. It was like a green tunnel, flecked with sunlight. "How's your pace?" she said. "A bit too fast," I said. "I thought so," she said. I slowed down. I ran through the green tunnel, feeling safe and calm and free. I was aware of the therapist's gentle touch and her presence, even though I could not see her. Time passed. I sensed that the therapy session was drawing to a close. "What's coming up for you now?" the therapist said. "I'm worried that we're running out of time," I said. "I don't want to go. I want to stay here. But I know I have to leave." "Yes," she said, "that's what's happening now."

Had it been possible, I would never have left the green tunnel, the feeling of running through it, not too fast, not too slow, just right, one step after another, surrounded by the trees. The session ended. I stood from the armchair.

Months passed. My emotions cycled between panic and despair. Sometimes it was hard to tell where the fear stopped and the heavy sadness began. It was hard to tolerate even a single waking minute. My mind fled to a million imaginary horizons in a search for sanctuary.

My first thoughts of suicide had a frightening and alien quality. Picture the effort entailed in solving a difficult puzzle, a Rubik's Cube, say, and the moment when you reach a point of frustration, ready to give up, only the Rubik's Cube is your own mind, and giving up means you have to kill yourself. Before long I thought about killing myself many times every single day, and then every hour, and then all the time, until the idea of self-annihilation became the background of every single other thought and feeling and memory in my awareness, like the air surrounding my body. My mind wore down from constant, unbidden contemplation of self-execution, an inner violence that eroded any defense against its murderous intention. The idea of oblivion flashed into my awareness like an empty sky above a distant mountain, as if death were a kind of sanctuary beyond the horizon of the living, a safe place I could run to, the next frontier on the journey that had taken me from England to California. *But kill myself? No. It will hurt. And if I die, I'm not going to the Land of the Dead. My body will rot in the ground. There will be nothing left of me at all. Just the sorrow of everyone I leave behind.*

Miriam and I joined her mother and stepfather on vacation in Hanalei on the Hawaiian island of Kauai. She had had enough. We spoke of divorce. Her parents understood that our marriage was on the verge of dissolution. They had heard that I was depressed. No one recognized the severe nature of my illness, which at the time I felt powerless to put into words.

"I don't want to leave you," said Miriam. "But you're sad *all the time*. I don't know what to do. I want to have kids. I know you said you did. Or do. But I don't know if that's what you really want anymore. I don't know what you want."

Earth seemed to conspire to keep me alive. The island manifested marvels of almost comic-book images of natural enchantment. One afternoon I paddled out in giant surf and looked back toward the shore. A rainbow formed above a tall green mountain. Giant waves crashed all about me. I wondered if the surf was big enough to guarantee death by drowning. A double rainbow formed above the mountain.

That evening I found a book of Buddhist scripture on the bedside table in our rental home. I opened the book to a random page, in a search for comfort. I found a passage that addressed the fate of a person who elects to die by suicide. Such a person would not be reborn in the realm of Buddhas or human beings or even the lowest animals, the book informed me. Such a person would be condemned to inhabit a hell realm for as many eons as there were grains of sand in the Ganges. I put the book down and laid my head on the pillow. I closed my eyes and tried to imagine a trillion eons in a hell realm, and I tried to ponder whether being in hell that long would be any worse than the torment that already afflicted me. I remembered meeting Miriam and the joy and hope I once had felt in being with her. Now our marriage lay in ruins. I had only myself to blame, I thought. I lay in bed aware of the hell where my mind used to be and the impossibility of expressing such torment in language. I understood that Miriam was angry. I understood that Miriam was sad. I understood myself to be the principal cause of those feelings in Miriam. I wished that I could say something. Long ago I would have spoken. But no more. Not that I wished to defend myself. Or to tell her she was wrong. Or that it was going to get better. Because it wasn't. She was right. There was no defending it, this lump of flesh I'd turned into. Nothing I could think to say. Not only about me or her. Or the rights or wrongs of being sad or mad. About anything. I could hear her crying. "I married a zombie," she said, in between sobs. And it was true. I'd become a zombie. Knowing this didn't make me sad. Or not any sadder. I'd sunk to the sadness floor. There was nowhere lower to go. I wasn't a person anymore. No, if I could speak, I would have said, *Miriam, you're not wrong. I'm so sorry. Sorry this happened. Sorry I turned into a zombie. Sorry the man you remember has gone and this is what I am now. Sorry, sorry, sorry.*

I STOOD BY THE window. It was gray outside. There was an immense silence into which I had fallen. I couldn't move. I couldn't speak. I had no thoughts. My sole emotion was fear. I didn't want to go. I didn't want to stay. It was gray outside. I stood by the window.

There are no words for madness. There have never been words for madness. Call it a crack-up or a nervous breakdown and you face an identical barrier. I don't dismiss endeavors to rid our language of stigmatizing labels. It is good that people of conscience avoid the bad old labels—words like *psycho* and *schizo* and *bonkers* and *nuts* and *loony* and *crazy*, the terms by which those of us with turbulent minds have been marked since the dawn of time as emotional lepers. Neither do I disparage the giant accomplishments of the mind sciences with their nomenclature for the myriad forms in which psychological distress can manifest. I am talking about a different problem. All the foregoing words describe madness from the outside. It is important to have objective descriptions. We have to call it *something*. Language is a function of reason. To put experience into words, the mind turns signals into symbols. Something seen or heard or felt becomes a kitty or a cupcake, an echo or a sigh. You can understand this sentence because you and I share a capacity for our eyes to absorb the symbolic patterns that form the words *you* and *can* and *understand* and *this* and *sentence* and process electrophysical signals from the optic nerve via the occipital lobe and the five layers of visual cortex into meaning. For perceptions at the outer frontier of experience, we can reach for a comparison. It was like *this*, we say. It was like *that*. But madness isn't like this or that. Madness resembles nothing except madness. It brooks no comparison—tending to serve, by contrast, as a descriptor of other things, if we want to dismiss something as nonsensical. I could say that madness is like getting pummeled by a giant ocean wave. I could say that it resembles the feeling of falling through space, the rush of fear, the awareness that there's no way out. You are going five fathoms down to the Kingdom of Poseidon. Well, madness is nothing like that. Waves come and go. Relax. Any second now, you'll figure out which way is up again, push from the sand, and make it to the surface. Then you'll breathe again. That kind of fall you can put into words because it's made of something you can see and touch and feel, a chaos of air and water. Madness disrupts something much more fundamental, the very medium in which things like air and water show up to us: consciousness. That is why there are no words for madness. Madness disrupts the foundation of communicability that language presupposes. And that is why it hurts so much. Your suffering is incommunicable, so you suffer it alone.

It was gray outside. I stood by the window.

"YOU COULD DIE," said our couples therapist, Thelma, observing my wretched demeanor on the couch one evening, mute and shivering, swaddled in a blanket, anesthetized by another ocean beating. "You need to go to Langley Porter."

A mental hospital. I had heard of it. Who knew what dark sorcery occurred there. The prospect of confinement was frightening. And yet I sensed my need for it, for some external structure to fold around me. Perhaps that meant walls. I imagined the feeling of them. I imagined a human chrysalis, a cocoon containing all the broken bits of me, holding those pieces until they grew together and were transformed. A couple of days earlier Miriam had said, "I wish I could take you someplace." I was in her arms, crying, as usual. "Like an island," she said, "a place where you'd be safe. Somewhere you wouldn't need to worry about anything."

When I imagined the asylum, I felt a measure of solace. But I also felt afraid. Once inside a psych ward I would need to relinquish any pretense of normality. I would be one of those unfortunates mocked and shunned as psycho, schizo, bonkers, nuts, bananas, crazy, loony, mental, crackers, or wacko, a designation that, like the literal brands on the skin that had marked the insane in medieval times, could never be removed. Transit across that threshold would incur a permanent mark of inferiority—a secret about which I could never speak a word.

The consequences of others knowing I had been there would presumably be ruinous. One part of this marginalization, I imagined, would be overt: jobs, for instance, I would never have. But I anticipated the worse part would be covert: whispers and odd glances from people who thought less of me or in whom I inspired pity; the judging gaze of the people who now saw me as broken; the gossip I'd never hear but whose inferred presence I would have to tolerate in my imagination. *Remember Jason? You know he totally lost it, right? Yeah . . . there was always something weird about that guy . . .* I would need to remain silent about it forever. In the country's de facto caste system, it seemed to me, mental patients got lumped together with junkies and prisoners and pedophiles among the American untouchables. Yet along with this dread I yearned for a period of respite—a place of refuge. I remember one time looking up monasteries online. I found the application page for one of them. You could not enter the monastery with ongoing mental illness, the document stated. I couldn't become a monk. And I knew the island of which Miriam had spoken existed only in her mind. I wanted a place where life could stop. I imagined something like a nineteenth-century sanitorium high in the Alps, the kind of place to where consumptive poets retreated in the terminal phase of their illness, a place where poems were written in fresh mountain air above a panoramic vista. But my imagination also summoned more horrifying specters of the asylum: there would be electric shocks to the brain and a straitjacket for misbehavior, like in *One Flew Over the Cuckoo's Nest*, I assumed. In sum, the prospect of psychiatric confinement inspired me at once with fear and desperate yearnings. Maybe, I thought, the shrinks would strap me to a table, or imprison me in a barrel of eels, as in the days of yore. But maybe what they offered would be instead a place of sanctuary, the type of healing refuge whose ideal version as a magic island Miriam's words had summoned in my sad and frightened mind.

BALL. BOOK. FLAG. Those were the three things the nurse told me to remember.

"Do you know where you are?" she said.

"In the hospital," I said. "In San Francisco, California."

"Do you know what day of the week this is?" she said. "What month and year? The number of the month?"

"Near the end of January 2005," I said. "Maybe Thursday."

"That's right," she said. "Can you tell me the name of the US president?" she said. "Or maybe a fairer question for you would be, who is the British prime minister?"

"Bush is president," I said. "Blair is the British PM."

"Okay. Now can you try something for me?"

"Yes," I said.

"I want you to count backward by seven from one hundred."

I performed my arithmetic task per the instructions of the nurse. "Ninety-three . . . eighty-six . . . seventy-nine . . ."

"What would you like me to put down," she said, "voluntary or involuntary?" There were potential merits to involuntary admission, she explained. My insurance company, she said, might be more inclined to pay the bill for an involuntary admission. The inpatient ward was reserved for the most serious forms of mental illness, one marker of which was that the patient didn't want to go to the hospital. A voluntary admission implied that I was making a choice in my own best interest. From such a voluntary decision it could be inferred that I retained the capacity to exercise the faculty of reason—emblematic of sanity—in which case I wasn't that sick after all.

I considered the logic of her question. It had the nuance of a riddle. Was my will to act against my will, she had essentially asked me. I didn't know how to answer. To speak at all seemed to be something which by definition I was choosing. The concept of involuntary admission summoned images of madmen in straitjackets. *He was taken to the madhouse*: Who'd say yes to that? Of my two bad choices I picked the one confirming that I had indeed made a choice. I would take the risk of a giant medical bill. But it would leave me with something that money couldn't buy: the knowledge that I had chosen my own direction.

I SAT ON A gurney. A large man in a dark uniform with a gun and a badge stood guard beside me. "You can lie down if you want to," he said. It was the middle of the afternoon. I wasn't tired. I had sustained no physical injury necessitating bed rest. I did not understand the reasons for my placement on the gurney. *Perhaps I am supposed to lie down.* Time passed. "You wanna stay there while I wheel you up to the unit?" said the guard. "No," I said, "I can walk." I stood. He took me to the elevator. I could sense no malice directed from the guard toward me. Yet upon entering the hospital I was aware of my transformation in the surveillance of those who ran the place from person into patient, subject into object. *This one seems harmless, but with the crazies you never know*, I could imagine the guard thinking. The elevator reached the fourth floor. From the elevator the guard led me down the hall and inside the ward, and then he locked the door behind me.

The One and the Many

I reach the bottom of the long descent. I follow the trail as it flattens and continues through the trees for a little while until I can see a white gravel path ahead of me, leading out of the trees into a clearing. There are a couple of people by the side of the trail—the first sign of human life I've seen in hours. They clap and whoop as I run by. I must be approaching the mile-10 aid station: Stephen Jones.

Run a 10K or even a road marathon and the received wisdom says: Keep going. Slow down and walk for a bit if you need to, no worries. Likely you'll pass tables now and then with friendly, generous people handing out little cups of water or energy drink. Drink it. Thank the friendly, generous people. Keep going till the finish line. This can work for 6 miles or 13 miles or even 26.2 but if you go beyond the border of the recognizable universe where runs still finish in a single calendar day and travel into Freaky Land, soon enough you run up against certain facts of your biology. You got to the start line from a longer path that began billions of years ago in the Archaean ocean, the single-celled life-forms that turned into the fish that flapped on the land that stood on two legs that wandered across Earth that turned into the grizzled ultra-runner, a person with a history and a mind and complicated thoughts but who in essence is still just a bunch of cells, a chemical entity that needs replenishing with ingredients from outside itself. Water. Food. Aid stations.

I can feel my brain shift gears. My mind's still in the high country, letting thoughts and feelings and memories run wherever their fancy takes them. But now I need to stop. Think. Plan. Decide. Because there are so many choices to be made! I'm standing in front of a table full of little paper plates. One is loaded with peanut butter sandwiches, another with sections of banana. I see cookies and candies, chips and cups of Coke and ginger ale. And that's not all, oh no! There are pickles and boiled potatoes and quesadillas and watermelon. Up in the high country, everything flowed into a single choiceless dreamy stream of sight and sound and breath and feeling and wondering and remembering: the many became one. But now I need to wake up. Choose. Carve the one back into many. Split perception into pieces. Behold the magnificent bounty! Verily, the gods and race organizers have smiled upon me and blessed me with this harvest, for they are wise and powerful and I a humble ultrarunner before the tasty morsels showered from the heavens in this sprawling smorgasbord.

Maybe I should eat the chips first, then drink the ginger ale . . . Or should I start with the ginger ale? So hard to know. And yet I must take action, ignorant though I may be. And beyond the choice of food, so many other tasks now face me. I must refill my water bottles. Apply sunscreen. Pack enough food for the twenty miles ahead. Dowse my head in ice water—it's boiling hot now. I shuffle about, picking up a boiled potato, refilling my water bottles, eating something else, drinking, eating again, conscious of my regression, of managing my tasks with the disorganized quality that can be observed in a tired kindergartner sorting Legos of variable dimensions into plastic bins—which is to say that I get my job done in the end and all the kind helpers applaud me when I pack up my satchel and wave bye-bye and run along to play. I like to run! Running is fun in the hot, hot sun!

III

Venus

Heat

The trail leads back into the forest and heads uphill. *Onward*. Running, you always look forward. You have to. This feeling now, seeing the trees, planting the right pole, then the left, knowing I'm getting somewhere, must be the absolute polar opposite of how I used to feel, circling around in my head, going nowhere.

The mountain summer heat is scorching. I can tell from the position of the sun overhead and the glare of the light against the white gravel path on the way out of the checkpoint toward the trailhead. But some of the normal signals are missing. You can't necessarily discern the heat from how you *feel*. Under extreme conditions, the signals get harder to read. The air's so dry in the mountains the sweat vaporizes so fast you don't even feel it on your skin. You don't always experience thirst. It takes a steady fluid intake to stay hydrated. You learn over the years to spot the early warning signs. The way your mouth dries up. A vague overall feel of the forward effort getting harder. The body is crying out, *I am thirsty*, but using a different language than the one you're used to. It must be in the high 70s now, a few hours after I left Stephen Jones. I'm almost out of water, running on an exposed stretch of trail with the sun baking down on me, breathing dry and dusty air that parches my lips and builds into a weary depletion that doesn't feel like thirst but which I hear as the speech of my shriveled cells, crying out for a drink. The body under stress speaks its own special language. You might think that a thirsty body would cry, *Water!* But instead it says, *I'm tired. I want to stop. This is stupid. I didn't train hard enough for this.* You learn to turn your attention to this voice and listen to the basic need that in its cranky and whiny way it's trying to communicate. I get it. *Don't worry—I'll find water.*

I can hear the trickle of a creek on the other side of a little mound on the left side of the trail. It looks like an easy scramble up no more than about twenty feet and then down the other side of the mound to the creek. A couple of runners overtake me. I'm not sure I know why they don't bother stopping. Either they didn't notice the creek or they're not low on water, or they figured it's too much hassle to climb the mound when there's likely an easier spot to access the creek farther down the trail. It's possible they've studied the map with a level of focus and rigor that's made them certain about where that next, easier spot is down to its exact GPS coordinates. If they've geeked out on the maps to that degree, good for them. If they're blowing past this awkward refill spot because they still have plenty of water, that makes sense. If they missed this spot, too bad. But if they're low on water and planning on running farther in the hope or expectation that they'll soon get somewhere better, in my experience of these adventures that's not a good call. Maybe the easier spot is ten minutes away. Maybe it doesn't exist. Then you're running on empty for miles, until the next aid station. By the time you reach water, you might notice your fatigue or a headache, but what you won't notice is the depletion deep on the inside, things you can't feel yet, hidden stresses in the basic structures underpinning life, which have a nasty habit of compounding on themselves and in the end leading to a breakdown. You've crossed a border into a different physiologic state—a whole different physical country, even. Bad things happen there. You can only go there if you know what you're doing, and have a plan to get back home again, or if someone's available to help you.

I scramble over the mound and down to the creek. I take off my shoes and socks and soak my dusty, hot, and bloated feet in the cold alpine water. It . . . feels . . . *so* . . . *good*. The instant my feet come out of the tight little feet prisons called shoes that they've been living in for the past six hours and dunk them underwater, the chill is such a tonic for all their angry inflammation, I can almost hear them saying thank you. I take out my ultraviolet-light water-purifying device, a fountain-pen-size plastic rod, stick it into one of my water bottles, press its postage-stamp-size rubber ON switch, and wait sixty seconds until the little smiley face comes on to tell me that my water is now pure. *Forty-eight . . . forty-nine . . . fifty . . .* It feels like an eternity. A frowny face appears. My water is impure! I try again. *Fifty-eight . . . fifty-nine . . .* smiley face. Now for the second bottle.

I soak my legs underwater. After all the hours of pounding on the trail, every muscle, joint, ligament, and tendon from my navel to my pinky toe has already taken quite a beating. In a run that lasts a few hours or even a whole day, I wouldn't normally indulge in this regimen of cold therapy. It wouldn't be worth the time. Barring a broken ankle, my thought in response to almost every conceivable hobble, owie, ache, or boo-boo—I believe those are the correct medical terms—is to keep on keepin' on and witness the natural magic of a moving organism spontaneously restoring itself to harmony, to *run it off,* as they say, and take care of any lingering aftereffects the morning after. But I can't do that here. Tomorrow I'll still be running. And the next day. And the day after that. And maybe the day after that. Twinges can turn into nerve damage, aching knees into a kind of agony you can't ignore.

What goes for muscles and tendons goes for everything else in the ultrarunner's body and mind. Avoid taking care of blisters and they turn into bleeding wounds. Skip stretching out tight calves and they turn into horrible cramps. Skimp on food and you wind up woozy and horizontal somewhere, wondering where you went wrong. All of this is, if not preventable, at least predictable and to some extent manageable if you take care of little problems before they spiral into big ones. I climb across the rocks to the side of the creek where I've left my shoes. I can feel how after the cold soak my legs feel more limber. I dry my feet with a bandanna and put on fresh, clean socks. Then I put my shoes back on and climb over the mound and back down to the trail. This whole excursion to get water and soak my legs and feet and change socks must have taken thirty minutes, maybe even longer. But it was so worth it. I might as well have had a leg transplant from someone ten years younger. As I run down the trail, I can't remember ever moving before with quite this same sense of strength and flow and freedom.

English Male, Disheveled

I woke to the sound of an old man snoring. He had the comatose look of a man sheltered like Rip Van Winkle in oblivious shut-eye to the horrors of the waking world for the entire preceding century, the lucky bastard. Consciousness: what a burden.

"Get up, boys. It's breakfast time," said a nurse, entering the room. In the bed next to Rip Van Winkle was a bearded man in a biker jacket, reading *Harry Potter and the Prisoner of Azkaban*. He had read the book six times in a row, he said. By the time he got to the end of the book, he couldn't remember the beginning. But he was goddamn lucky he could still focus on a book, he said, on account of there being no TV in the room and not much else to do. "If we put TVs in the rooms, you guys would never come out," said the nurse who'd shown me around the night before, in between letting me stash my spare underpants in my cubby and confiscating my shoelaces.

I went to the bathroom. I washed myself in the shower with a little bar of hospital soap. There was this weird chemical scent in the shower from the kind of cheap disinfectant they use in jails and public schools in poor neighborhoods and other places where people are trapped and powerless. The smell of confinement.

I went to the dining room and took my place at a table upon which was laid a plastic tray of inedible food in a seat across from the Prisoner of Azkaban. I ate some oatmeal and drank some decaffeinated coffee.

I followed the other patients to a little room at the back of the unit. I sat on a couch facing a window through which gray sky and eucalyptus trees were visible. There were about ten of us patients in the room, many still in blue hospital pajamas. The Prisoner had the worst headache in history, he said, from his latest round of electroconvulsive treatment, or ECT. In addition to the plot of Harry Potter, he had no memory of the month prior to his hospitalization. Yet now he wanted to kill himself only a couple of times a day instead of every waking millisecond, he said. Better to lose his memory than his three score years and ten. The therapist gave us notepads and told us about how molehills were often misconstrued as mountains and asked us to write down our molehills, and I tried to think of what my molehills might be, but all I could picture were the actual moles that once left little mounds of dirt in the garden at Cannon Road, a whole bunch of them, appearing overnight like magic, in this amazing regular pattern. "Let's hear about some of those molehills," said the therapist, and a young Hispanic woman said that the police had taken her to the hospital because she wanted to drown her baby in the bathtub, and until she took the pills she thought she had turned into La Llorona, the ghost of a lady who killed her kids after her husband left her and then was condemned to wander the Earth in search of her lost children for the rest of time.

Late that morning a young woman in a white coat found me in my room and introduced herself in the perkiest tone I had heard in rather a long while. "Hello, Mr. Thompson! I'm Dr. Browning, one of the psychiatry residents," she said. "I'll be the main doctor taking care of you."

She saw a *slender English male, disheveled, good eye contact, speech normal in volume.* I saw a doctor several years my junior, a person who'd likely had all her shit together since kindergarten and aced every test and been kind to dogs and spent her gap year helping orphans and had her choice of fancy medical schools and specialties but picked the really hard thing, the hospital where half the patients wanted to die instead of go on living, or wondered if perhaps they were already dead; a person who stood poised upon the threshold into grown-up life while I was still singing karaoke in a toy store; a person who surely looked at a loser like me and wondered what had gone wrong with him, and along with her pills and notepad pulled out lines like *That sounds really hard* to disguise her pity.

WHAT TIME IS NOW? The present moment has a duration. Listen to the notes *do, re, mi* with the sounds close together and your mind binds them in a musical phrase: *do-re-mi*. Separate the sounds by a long gap and you hear them as disconnected notes: *do*, pause, *re*, pause, *mi*. Separate the sounds by only a millisecond and they pile on top of one another, sounding as if they are being heard simultaneously. These upper and lower thresholds of perception define the borders of *now*. As the nineteenth-century German philosopher Edmund Husserl described in his writings on the psychology of time perception, *now* has three parts: an echo of the moment just gone, the immediate present, and an anticipation of the moment to come.[8] You don't experience a stream of disconnected moments: the present always enfolds both the time just gone and the expected time just ahead.

But there's no bright dividing line between the feeling of *now* and its recession into *the past*. The present is elastic, shrinking in emergency to a tiny sphere, expanding in reverie or reminiscence to enclose echoes of times past. Trauma and tragedy can split the flow of time awareness into a feeling of *before* and *after*, as if the world prior to the instant of disaster and the world that succeeded it are forever and irreparably severed, even if *before* in literal terms was only yesterday.

I sat down at the piano. I put my fingers on the keys. I hadn't played since my teens, but the memory of the major scales was still in my hands. I watched the fingers of my right hand press the keys in succession from middle C up an octave—*do-re-mi-fa-sol-la-ti-do*—and then back down again. I placed the little finger of my left hand an octave below middle C and then both hands moved together. Up and down I went, from *do* to *do*, feeling the rhythm become smoother, the pressure and velocity of each keystroke more even. I felt a sort of solace in sensing how each finger's movement always matched its corresponding sound, the right thumb's *do*, the index finger's *re*, the *mi* of the middle finger. Soon I switched from C major to D major, and then E major, F major, G major, A major, and B major, and as I listened to the sounds climbing up and then down again, the circular monologue in my head went quiet. I experienced the notes of each scale forming a kind of whole, how *re* contained *do*'s echo and the anticipation of *mi*, how the sound just gone and the sound still to come, though nonexistent, had a kind of presence, the way now spilled over into portions of time past and the yet-to-be. I stopped playing and went for lunch. As the circling sound of *do-re-mi* fell silent, all I could hear was the loop of sad and frightened thinking in my mind.

A NURSE LED ME into a tiny windowless room. "Hello, I'm Dr. Hewitt, the attending," said the woman who greeted me. She had long black curly hair and the somber air of a serious person put in charge of a dismal situation. She wore a Timex Ironman waterproof watch with stopwatch and lap-counting functions. "Tell me how long you've been feeling depressed," she said. The doctor listened to me as I spoke, scribbling notes now and then. "Your depression has lasted longer than most," she said. "But depression is a finite phenomenon."

In the evening I sat in the dayroom, listening to other patients as they spoke.

It was almost impossible for me to speak. But I could listen. And to do so was to shift the focal point of my awareness outside myself: for a moment my painful inner monologue fell silent.

"I've never not been sad or scared," said a middle-aged woman with short brown hair. "Sometimes the sadness is worse, other times fear. Sometimes I'm sad but not afraid or scared, and other times I'm sad and scared both at once. But whichever it is I feel terrible, all the time. Except when I'm sleeping. I do get good sleep, so I'm lucky, I suppose—I know there are lots of folks like us who don't. Yeah, I'm lucky. I have an apartment and this little job in a store. I think about all those poor people out on the street, you know. I have it so much easier. But I think that and then I'm even sadder and it all just seems pointless. Life, I mean. Really, no point. Nothing and nobody to live for. No husband, no kids, no friends. And it's not like I do some job that makes any difference to anyone. I work in a stationery store, for chrissakes. But I guess Mom and Dad would miss me. They're old now. So I need to wait. But it's hard, you know? 'Cause I think I've really tried. I've been good. I take the pills. Never miss a single one. Never miss a single therapy appointment. I must have done 'em all, every type of pill and therapy. But everyone has limits, right? Can't I go? Maybe Mom and Dad would understand. But I worry it would hurt them. People always say, 'Hold on. It gets better.' Like it's this religion we're supposed to believe in: It Will Get Better. But I'm not sure I have the willpower left to believe in anything. I'm tired. So tired. I wanna keep trying. I do. But the word that comes to mind is *cynical*. I get cynical. I wanna think one day I'll be happy. Someday, somehow, somewhere over the rainbow. But I'm running out of energy. I'm not sure how much longer I can keep on going." The Shopkeeper paused. Then she said, "I don't know if any of this makes sense to you." "It does," I said. "You know something," said the Shopkeeper, "you're a great listener."

"HOW ARE YOU FEELING this morning, Mr. Thompson?" said Dr. Browning, entering my room. Several days had passed since my arrival on the ward. I was in a state of undress. The doctor averted her gaze as I put on my shirt. "Any suicidal thoughts at all?"

Mr. Thompson—her formal salutation induced a feeling of distance between us, constraining any capacity I might have had to respond with candor.

Nothing had changed since the door on the locked unit had closed behind me five days before, except my being stuck inside. If I went back outside, I'd still be me, the world's worst worrywart. But I would be me outside. I could go get drilled by giant waves. Eat whatever I wanted. Shave without a nurse in surveillance. All that being inside did was put the world's worst worrywart somewhere with nothing to do. Being inside just added boredom to all the worry. *How am I feeling, Dr. Browning? Much worse, if you really want to know. And I know you do want to know. You're really asking. It's not some bullshit question. You find out people's feelings for a living! I know it's supposed to help, having another person know how you're feeling. Trust no one, keep the secrets, stuff it all inside where no one else can see . . . Isn't that how I've lived my whole life? And look where it got me. So I guess I should tell you, if I want you to help me. That would mean saying,* Yes, Dr. Browning, lots and lots of suicidal thoughts. One every minute! *But then you'd know I'm not getting better, and you wouldn't let me out of here. Then I'd be stuck inside. And I don't see how that would help. Show my insides to you on the outside so I don't feel so alone there, and you'll keep me locked up in this place.*

Unlike an illness of the liver or the lung, an affliction of the mind is much less conspicuous in any medical scan than the credulous exaggeration of rainbow-colored brain maps in popular science articles typically tends to imply. In reality, the doctors had my words to go on and not much else. They could listen to my silence. They could listen to what I didn't say. They could observe my movements on the ward and interactions with other patients and from this paucity of data they would infer a picture of my mind and in particular my stance upon a single question: Did I want to live or die? How I yearned for the kind of trust in the care of another that would make it possible for me to answer this question with candor. But if I let Dr. Browning know my true thoughts and feelings, I feared it would turn her from doctor into captor. "I'm feeling fine now," I said. "Much better, actually. I'd like to go home soon if that's all right." *I have her fooled.* She saw right through me. "If patient decides to leave AMA,"* she wrote in my medical chart that night and I read years later, "strongly consider 5150."**

---

* Against medical advice
** In section 5150 of a 1968 law created by the State of California, the Lanterman-Petris-Short Act, police officers and county officials are given the legal authority to involuntarily detain for up to seventy-two hours a person who, "as a result of a mental health disorder, is a danger to others, or to himself or herself, or gravely disabled."

One morning I found a man with a bandaged forearm sitting at the piano. I watched his fingers flurry across the keys to produce a sound like a maestro in a concert hall. The music started loud and fast and angry and then got slow and quiet.

"That's incredible," I said. "What is it?"

He glanced over his shoulder to reply. "Holst," he said. "*The Planets.*"

"I thought you needed a whole orchestra for that," I said.

"Yeah, it's something I put together," he said.

"You must be a genius," I said.

"Whatever," he said with a shrug.

I listened to Holst until he finished playing, and then I returned to my circular walk around the ward.

YOU CAN'T THINK YOUR way out of severe depression. Indeed, a certain kind of runaway thinking is one of depression's defining characteristics. A group of brain regions connected to learning, memory, and the experience of self-awareness, called the default mode network (DMN), goes haywire as the thinking mind turns in on itself. Look at the neuroimaging maps from a person with major depression and you'll see the signs of neural signals sprinting up and down the paths between the interconnecting regions that constitute the DMN like a panicky runner lost in a labyrinth of forking forest trails.[9] But that part of the brain goes quiet when a person disengages from the inner world of thinking and remembering and engages in their five senses and the outside world. You can't turn off the DMN—remove those regions of the brain and you'd no longer know or remember things; it's part of what makes human consciousness so special. But the sphere of human consciousness is larger than reason. Humans are also embodied, feeling, sensing beings—creatures who see and touch and hear, who love and hate and fear, who feel shame and compassion and joy. This embodied and feeling dimension of consciousness is neither more nor less important than the thinking mind. Being human means doing both, finding a way to think, feel, and move between these elements of the mind and integrate them.

I circled the corridor of the ward lost in thought: worrying, remembering, contemplating one pole of something binary and then the other, pondering where I should live and what I should do for a living, considering whether or not I was ready to be a father, feeling my mind form knots with every terrified rotation, sensing that despite my wish to put an end to this ceaseless cogitation it would not end until one pole of any binary made more sense in a final and irrevocable form—resolving, for instance, that California was doubtless superior to England, yet in the instant of determining California as superior, feeling the loss of England as a possibility, forever sealed off and now unreachable, and then thinking, *No, the answer must be England,* but then feeling California likewise vanish into oblivion. As my thoughts continued to circle in this manner, I walked around the unit, reflecting on my awareness that my mind had run in precisely this intolerable form for every second of every minute not only since that morning but for what felt like many months if not years. Something had gone wrong in my brain. My disturbance felt so profound that I assumed it had to be permanent. How I wished for something or someone to help me! *Please, oh God, please help me, won't you?* But I didn't believe in God. I didn't believe in anyone—least of all myself. It was hard to see the point of carrying on the charade of hoping for recovery or rescue. I was alone. Abandoned. No one was listening. No one had ever been listening. If anyone was ever going to do anything to put an end to all my worrying and all my ceaseless oscillation between this thing or that thing or this thing or that thing and help me run away from my unbearable, unspeakable, unending runaway thinking, it was me, only me, just me.

Gravity

Trees. Everywhere I look, trees. A switchback fifty feet ahead. *Left, right, left right. Plant one pole, then the other. Huff, puff, get it done. Reach the turn. Go right. What's ahead? Yup: more trees. Another switchback, a couple hundred feet ahead. Left, right, left right. Huff, puff, right, left, plant the right pole then the left one, breathe in, breathe out, huff-puff, get it done. Reach the turn. Guess what? More trees. . . .*

It's been going on like this forever. I haven't been slogging uphill through the forest since the beginning of time. It just *feels* that way. Judging by the course profile, I'm somewhere in the middle of a two-thousand-foot climb. At some point I'll reach the top of the climb, then head all the way down again to the mile-30 aid station, by a little town near the lake's northwestern shore, Tahoe City. But it's hard to translate numbers that land in my mind like pure abstraction—two thousand feet—into grunts and fatigue and the reality of a destination beyond the limits of what I can see right in front of me, or expect to see twenty or ten or even five of these turns ahead, at some point becoming *here*.

In theory I could stop, look at the satellite map on a GPS app called Gaia, which the race organizers asked us all to download, so I'd know exactly where I am. But it seems like too much effort. Not to mention, sometimes it feels like I'm better off *not* knowing. When you know how far it is to the end, and there's still a long way to go, that can be a tough kind of knowledge to bear. Fixate on some future that isn't here yet, and the present is a bad place to be. Drop that fixation, and the present is neither good nor bad. It just *is*.

So that's what I end up doing. I drop all thoughts of ever getting to the top. I focus only on the bit of trail I can see directly ahead, until the next turn. *Huff, puff, right, left, plant the right pole then the left one, breathe in, breathe out . . .*

IT'S SWELTERING NOW. It must be in the 80s. I come across this guy sitting down, slumped against a tree. He's red in the face, silent, and dazed looking. In ultras, especially the really long ones like this, runners have to think of themselves as de facto first responders. Tahoe City must be about six miles away; four miles of that is steep uphill. Move at a solid pace and the next aid is ninety minutes away, minimum. But this guy isn't moving at all. He's not gonna die. We're in the Sierra, not the Sahara. But there's more at stake than mortality statistics here. There's also the ethics of the thing. How we want to relate to one another. What sort of culture and community we want to have, our merry little band of sweaty freaks in trucker hats. Venus was the god of love. Humans are a social species, and love is the emotional gravity that keeps us together.

"How are you doing?" I say. "Not good," he says, shaking his head. His voice is hoarse, and his eyes have a disoriented look. "Whatcha need?" I say. He doesn't speak.

Having had my fair share of rough spots in long ultras, I understand that this man is having a hard time parsing a diffuse yet global sense of overwhelm into signals for specific tangible needs. Under ordinary conditions, when you're hot or thirsty, you *know* you're hot or thirsty, and you can easily separate those two perceptions as distinct. But after hours of intense exertion, those signals get harder to discern as dissociable needs—they start melding together into a vague overall awareness of reaching or appearing to exceed some safe upper threshold of What You Can Handle. *I can't do this*, you might think, or *I'm done*. But take stock of the situation, ask yourself, *When was the last time I drank something, or ate something, or ate something salty, or cooled my head down?* Then attend to the body's basic needs for food, water, or salt to ensure the water gets absorbed and the heat is regulated, and usually what happens is the diffuse sense of overwhelm resolves into awareness of a specific unmet need you've now succeeded in meeting. *I CAN do this!* you think. It takes practice to reach the point where you can read the signals by yourself. Everyone starts out like this, and I don't just mean runners. Once upon a time you were this teeny little thing that couldn't do anything. You didn't know you were hungry or thirsty or tired. You were just this cute little bundle of sensation. Someone else had to read the signals for you. *Oh, there, there, baby. Mama's here. Dada's here.* They had to have names for your needs, and know what to do.

I ask the runner by the tree if he's okay for water. "I'm out," he says, turning an empty bottle upside down. I'm almost out as well. There's about six ounces left in one of my bottles. But I do well in the heat. I've trained my body to handle extreme heat by doing things like ninety-minute runs in 100-degree weather in southern Mexico and push-ups in a sauna, so I figure I can manage the six miles to the mile-30 aid station down by the lake on three ounces of water. I pour half the contents of my water bottle into the man's bottle. "I'll tell them to expect you at the aid station," I say, making a mental note of the number on his race bib. He drinks the water and stands up. He begins to walk up the trail. I say goodbye to him and then I'm off again, hiking uphill through the trees.

I reach the top of the climb. The trail heads downhill. Not long now until I reach Tahoe City. It will be so good to see Miriam and my son and daughter. I can already picture their smiling faces, as if the feeling of being with them then has traveled back in time, so I'm feeling it right now. Sometimes the mind runs ahead of the body.

The Dark Age

I chased the other boys along the path from the tree near the pond toward the edge of the woods. I could hear myself panting. The pain in my chest was the worst agony. How I wished for it to stop! But there was no escaping it. Perhaps I could have pretended to be sick when I woke that morning. But Mum and Dad would never have believed me. They sent me to school even when I really had the flu. No, there was no turning back now. This was cross-country. It was going to hurt. That much was certain. The pain would go on for a very long time before the run was over. If I had any choice in the matter I wouldn't be here in this desperate scramble, feeling the acid burn in my legs and the panic of fighting for air with each heaving breath. I watched the phalanx of skinny, fast boys pull farther and farther ahead and then disappear in the trees while a wave of other runners passed me one by one, and I fought with all my might to hold my pathetic position somewhere near the back of the pack.

One evening in my final year at St. Peter's my mother had entered my room with a little brochure in her hand. There was a picture on the front of a giant building with a tall clock tower. "This is King Edward's," she said. "It's a private school. A place for clever boys. You'll take the entrance exam next month." I got into the back of our green Citroën 2CV. I looked at the fields through the window on the twelve-mile drive to Southampton. It felt like a world away. Sometimes on Saturdays we would go shopping at the big department stores there. After shopping, my parents would take us to La Margherita, an Italian restaurant, where we would have pizza and Coca-Cola and zabaglione. My father parked the car a few hundred feet from the gates of the school. The entire edifice of the school's south-facing aspect stood as barren as the monochrome illustration in the brochure. Inside, I joined a group of boys sitting at old wooden desks set in a geometric array in one of the classrooms. There were two little booklets on my desk. I opened the first one. It was the math portion of the exam. I raced through several pages of easy arithmetic problems. Then the questions got harder. I read something like "$2x = 4 + y$" and the instruction: "Solve for x when $y = 2$." Panic hit me as I struggled to interpret these alien concepts. I closed the math booklet, feeling my stomach turn somersaults. I opened the English exam. The examiners directed me to write. I wrote a story in the first person about a boy on holiday in Northern Ireland. "I wanted to climb Binnian," the story began. "My parents wouldn't let me. I decided to go there by myself. In the middle of the night I crept out of the house and went to climb the mountain. It was dark and hard to find my way. I reached the craggy summit and started back down the mountain. In the darkness of the trail, I wandered off a cliff and fell a thousand feet to my death below."

The Dark Age, Sebastian remembers calling those years: why that particular phrase came to his mind, he wasn't sure at the time, but there it was. For reasons that didn't make sense until much later, we stopped speaking to each other sometime around then, retreating to our bedrooms, in his words, like "solitary soldiers." It was certainly dark and cold when my father woke me on winter mornings. I got out of bed, shivering, and then put on my uniform and hurried downstairs, to find the cereal sitting in the milk and forming a mushy slop. I ate the cereal and downed a cup of orange juice. The milk curdled in my stomach. I felt sick. I put on my parka and left the house. I got in the back of our green Citroën. Dad drove me to the railway station. I walked onto the platform. I looked down the track, where the line stretched to a vanishing point in the distance, where a small black dot appeared and then expanded to become the front of the incoming train. The train entered the station with a roaring sound. I boarded the carriage and slid onto one of the blue upholstered seats near the heater. I felt warmer. At once the gas smell from the heater intensified my nausea. The train left the station. I looked through the window at the passing fields and meadows where the cows were still asleep. The countryside turned into gray and white factories and warehouses. The train went into a long, dark tunnel and emerged at Southampton Central station. I stepped from the railway carriage to the platform. The aroma of buttered toast wafted from the railway cafeteria, where slot machines chirped and shimmered. I followed some other boys in their dark blue uniforms up the stairs that led across a walkway to the other side of the tracks. I showed my ticket to the guard and left the station. In winter and spring it was often raining. By the time I'd walked the mile from the station to school my hair and clothes were soaked. I followed the road that led to the giant brick rectangle of King Edward's.

A huge green lawn extended from the gate on the street to a tall front door through which only the headmaster and teachers were permitted to enter or exit. I walked to the back, where a throng of boys in uniforms fluttered around a gray asphalt yard like a murder of crows. Among them strode the sixth formers, giant men seemingly double the size of me, bearing hardcover physics and Latin books in the crooks of their long arms, and others twice my width, massive shouldered and laughing like they ruled the place.

In morning assembly, we would sing the hymn "Our God, Our Help in Ages Past" by Sir Isaac Watts. It was the school anthem. Sir Isaac was right, I thought. God had helped us in ages past. But he was no use in ages present. I walked to 1B, one of the rooms for the younger pupils on the southern side of the ground floor. I took my seat at a wooden desk three rows back on the right-hand side. I sat shivering, my clothes still drenched from the rain. Mr. Butler, a man with curly brown hair and a suit jacket, entered the classroom. Everyone stood up when a teacher entered the room until they were told to sit down again. Mr. Butler read an alphabetical list of surnames from his light blue attendance book. He reached Thompson, and I said, "Yes, sir."

What were my instructions as Thompson at King Edward's? You may wear a sweater only in the winter—permissible colors are black and navy blue. Never remove the school tie, except for PE or Games—even upon exiting the gates during lunch and walking between school and the train station. You are a King Edward's pupil. You represent the school. You must maintain the uniform's integrity. Arrive at your form room no later than 8:45 a.m. Your group master may have information: listen to him. Lessons, with the exception of Tuesday, will begin at 9:00 a.m. Tuesday starts with assembly—you will sing hymns and listen to the speaker. There will be announcements: pay attention to them. At the sound of the bell, pick up your books and pencil case and find the classroom for the next period. You must carry your books in your hands—bags are forbidden. As a first-year you will take Mathematics, French, English, Latin, History, Geography, Science, Music, Art and Design, Religious Education, and Physical Education. Every day, with the exception of Wednesday, has four periods in the morning and three in the afternoon. Wednesday has five periods in the morning. Watch the Math teacher draw chalk equations on the blackboard. Listen to him speaking. Open your textbook to page whatever and do questions blah to blah. Calculate the highest common factor. Wait for the clock hands to say 9:15. Observe the rebels cackle and pratfall, the teacher grimace, the detentions administered to exterminate dissent. Calculate the lowest common denominator. Feel the weight of time already traversed since 9:00. Contemplate the vast expanse of Being until break time. Watch the clock hands reach 9:30. Experience each minute as an epoch in history. Witness each such era successively lengthen in duration. Hear the bell ring. Thank Lord Jesus for his mercy. Go to second period. Open *Histoires Illustrées* to a cartoon about a boy who steals some apples on a farm. Write a story about naughty little Pierre in the third-person perfect: *Il était une fois un petit garçon méchant appelé Pierre. Un jour, il a grimpé à un pommier. Soudain, le fermier est arrivé. "Oh mon Dieu!" a dit Pierre. Il s'est enfui aussi vite que possible.*[*] Wait for the bell. Feel an immense burden lifting. Follow the other boys to the mob by the tuckshop. Find a path through the melee to the window. Hold your money high above

---

[*]   *Once upon a time there was a naughty little boy called Pierre. One day, he climbed an apple tree. Suddenly, the farmer arrived. "Oh my God!" said Pierre. He ran away as fast as possible.*

your head. Yell for Mars or Twix, or Marathon or Maltesers, or Wispa or Bounty or Revels. Swap your coins for sweets. Suck each chocolate orb until your saliva dissolves it. Hear the bell signaling the end of morning break. Go back inside the school: your Revels now are ended.

Then came the wilderness of lunchtime. I would walk the playing field perimeter with Roland, a fellow choirboy, complaining about the futility of everything. The nuclear missiles had arrived in England. Outside the US military base at Greenham Common a group of women set up a permanent protest camp: the Greenham Common women, people called them. One time the women arrived in their thousands from all over Britain, joining hands in a giant circle that surrounded the base. But all the protests had come to nothing.

School was stupid, Roland and I agreed. They had rules for the sake of having rules. There was no rhyme or reason to any of them. Maggie Thatcher the Milk Snatcher was stupid. "There is no such thing as society," she once said in a speech. You're an individual, she said. Get a job, make loads of money, and shut your bloody mouth. Ronny Raygun was stupid. He loved the Milk Snatcher. He thought ketchup was a vegetable, and he believed that poor black women were driving Cadillacs in the ghetto. He came from Hollywood and thought he was still in a movie. He called the Soviet Union "the Evil Empire," as if Gorbachev was Darth Vader and he was Luke Skywalker. Church was stupid. Sometimes I'd remember how I'd believed in God and Jesus and all that rubbish when I was little, and it was hard to believe that silly kid and me were the same person. God was a fairy tale. I could see that now. You might as well pray to the Easter Bunny. Why I went through with Confirmation is hard to say. It was a way to meet girls, I suppose, at the youth club disco.

Rugby was stupid. PE was stupid. Sports Day was stupid. Roland would listen for a while, but then one day he ran and joined the Lads, the taller boys on the sports team with deep voices and girlfriends and mindless grins and not even the slightest fear of detention or failing grades or the fury waiting for them at home. "Pile on!" one of the Lads would yell, summoning Lads from all directions, who would leap onto one of their brethren and form a giant mass of squirming bodies on the ground, and as Roland's body joined the Lad pile, I left him there and followed the playing field perimeter on a path toward the library, where I would typically sit in the corner by the window and the radiator and disappear into Middle Earth or Fantasia until the bell rang and I went back to class and sat gazing at the blackboard and watched the minute hand on the clock and wished I had the power to propel it forward in motion with my mind.

The only things that weren't stupid were books and the inside of my own head. I had my own little kingdom up there. My thoughts ran wherever they wanted. Sometimes at Sunday mass, saying the Lord's Prayer, I would remember the feeling of believing in God's literal existence and marvel that something that had once felt so solid, no less basic to the structure of my perception than vision or hearing, could totally disintegrate. I couldn't remember exactly when I'd stopped believing. But now it was obvious: my thoughts were my own and nobody else's. I wasn't having conversations with God, Jesus, the Virgin Mary, Saint Peter, or Saint Maximilian. *It was me*: the experience of a conscious being. Thoughts of the past and the future, ideas of good and evil, imagination, reason and fantasy: all of it happened in my mind. I didn't know how. It was amazing, the way things showed up in awareness, but there was no reason to imagine a deity had put them there. Sometimes I noticed the gap between thoughts, the background sense of presence within which everything emerged, what it was like to have or be a mind. I noticed how it didn't seem to resemble any other thing, because it was the medium in which things themselves existed. It was like the air to a bird borne aloft, noticeable only through its disturbance, sudden pockets of low pressure that pulled the bird downward. It was with me in waking awareness and receded in dreams and vanished in deep sleep. It could be frightening, knowing I was alone there, that my thoughts were nobody else's. But I felt liberated too, knowing I was safe, that I could do anything I wanted there.

But it was lonely at lunchtime, pacing the playground boundary in silent contemplation, kicking a soda can from one end of the lawn to the other, making solo sorties to the sweetshop down the road, where the old lady behind the counter gave me a quarter of rhubarb-and-custards at half price with a smile of grandmotherly commiseration. I watched the other boys play their mindless games in the field and was overcome by a feeling of weariness. How busy they were with running and laughing, how pointless. I felt myself dwindling to a ghost. Perhaps the apocalypse had already happened, I thought. The bombs had already fallen all across Earth. Everything was burning. Nothing had survived. Not even time. The fire had sent a shock wave from the future to the past and burned me. I was nothing but a shadow on a wall.

I came to understand the imperative to relieve myself from my chronic feelings of loneliness and isolation. In the summer between my first and second years at the school, I traveled to Cornwall with the school choir. On the journey home an older boy in the bass section handed me a can of Carlsberg Special Brew. It was fabled to be the strongest beer in Britain. I took some sips and soon felt something dissolve within me and then the kind of ecstasy that comes along with a sudden relief from a long and agonizing pain. *I'm not afraid.* The fear was gone. I had not known of its existence. It was like I had lived my life until that moment with a mysterious headache, then realized I'd been wearing a hat that didn't fit me, and I took that hat off and felt the headache disappear. I looked around at the other boys and teachers in the bus and wondered if this fearless state might be how other people felt all or much of the time. I found myself giggling and singing and gazing out the window, learning that alcohol appeared to illuminate a basic need of which until then I hadn't been aware existed in me—the need to feel carefree and expansive and spontaneous and say or think things without being afraid of what might happen, of a judgment from God, whose existence I no longer believed in, or someone else, I didn't know.

And other than booze was wanking—masturbation—a delight I discovered in the bathroom of a boat on the English Channel during the choir tour in Denmark the following year, although it was a delight that I understood to be dirty: a Good Boy was not a wanker. One time I was sitting in the living room reading a novel whose blurb included the word *sex*, and observing me with the book, Mum took it from my hands and read the blurb and asked me if I knew what sex was, and I said yes, and that was the last time we ever discussed the topic. Not that knowing the word got me closer to anything like the act it signified. I could recall the little kid I once had been, playing kiss chase with the girls at St. Peter's, but now I would gaze at the girls at the far end of the train platform in the morning with their green uniforms and flicks of hair and callous smiles, and I yearned for them to notice me and wished for the touch of a warm hand and friendly eyes that met mine and saw me, but this never came to pass. Once at the Catholic youth club disco I noticed a girl called Ruth looking at me and not looking away, and I asked her to dance, and she said yes, and we stood swaying to the music, and I felt her squeeze my body closer to hers, and I pulled her even closer as I listened to the words of the song for the slow dance—"Arthur's Theme" by Christopher Cross—beneath the glittering disco ball, with Ruth in my arms, feeling that, yes, it was crazy, but true, I was caught between the moon and New York City, and I spent the next day singing her name throughout the house, but when I saw her again at a roller disco and we held hands and skated in circles around the room, my palms went clammy with sweat and I was too afraid to ask her to go out with me, so I got another boy to ask her for me, and she said no, and a dark cauldron of sorrow and rage then ignited inside me as I pictured myself decades in the future, a famous astronaut, sitting in my rocket ship surging through the troposphere at escape velocity and into orbit while sad old Ruth sat at home watching me on television, remembering the boy she'd spurned at the roller disco all those years before and ruing her terrible judgment.

I worked hard and rose to the top of my class. As I walked across the stage at the start of the next school year to receive my class award and a hardback copy of *Oliver Twist*, I felt a great swell of pride. *This nice feeling comes from being the best at something*, I thought. *I must finish first. Then I'll win prizes. Maybe one day I'll get into Oxford.*

Oxford: how I yearned to take up residence in this City of Knowledge! Achieve acceptance from this hallowed institution and I would be Someone. The significance of the place first hit me when Mum, Dad, Sebastian, and I visited the city a couple of years before. We walked through Radcliffe Square, a cobblestoned street surrounded by ancient gray stone buildings, in the center of which stood a domed structure, the Radcliffe Camera. We settled beneath a large tree in Christchurch Meadow to enjoy a picnic lunch. I lay down on the grass and stared at the leaves dancing in the wind. I felt the warmth of the sun on my face. A calm and peaceful feeling soaked through my body. If it were possible, I would have remained suspended in that state of reverie forever. It seemed to me that the calm feeling bore some relation to the antiquity of the buildings I had seen and the ancient knowledge in them. Oxford was a mystical place. It was here, among these medieval spires, I understood that some of the greatest minds in history—Erasmus, John Donne, Stephen Hawking—had thought their brilliant thoughts. Percy Shelley and Oscar Wilde had written masterpieces here. I had a feeling of awe that reminded me of how I felt looking at the images of Jesus and the Virgin Mary in the stained-glass windows in church when I was a little boy and still believed in God. Literature had become my religion. I didn't pray to Conrad or Dostoevsky or Milton, but the absorption I felt when reading books seemed to replicate the experience of contacting an intelligence beyond myself that kept me company and guided me.

I stopped making any kind of effort in PE. What was the point in running? My brain would get me prizes. My body was just the lump of flesh that carried my brain from PE to Chemistry and English, from Physics to Math and Music, from History to French to Latin. The following year some of the other boys started overtaking me in Science and Math. *I'm ordinary. Nobody.* I focused all my effort on the one class where I sensed no one else could touch me: English. By the time I was thirteen I must have read half the books on the living room shelves at home. When I was reading *Oliver Twist*, I felt like I was really inside Oliver's mind. Reading was magic. Read a book, and I got to know another human being on the inside, in the intimate way that I knew myself, but combined with a clearer sense of meaning, because in my own life things didn't always make sense in the moment, because I hadn't lived my whole life yet, only the little part that was *now*, and to really understand a story I had to see the whole—to know how everything turns out in the end when I looked back at how I got there from the beginning. In a book, I could see how a whole story fit together, from start to finish: how Oliver was born an orphan, for instance, and became a thief under the dubious care of the Artful Dodger, but then met the benefactor who adopted him and took him to a happy life in the countryside where he lived out the rest of his days.

The same year I started the school for clever boys, my mother finished her degree and got a teaching credential and started work at a nearby high school. She didn't last long in the job. She got a job in a different school. Then she changed jobs again. The job changes seemed innocuous at the time. Sometimes I felt sad or scared or lonely, but I saw no link between these feelings and the beginnings of more perplexing behavior in my mother, or the strange rules that applied in our home that I knew didn't apply in the homes of other boys. Sebastian once wrote up a list of guests for his forthcoming birthday party. He was turning ten or thereabouts. My mother crossed off the names of all the girls. "Why can't they come?" said Sebastian. "I don't want them to," said Mum. And that was that.

I had strange worries. One time I left my hockey stick on the train home. The prospect of telling my mother that I had lost the hockey stick was frightening. At the end of my second year I won the school poetry-writing prize. "My mother is dead," I wrote. "My father is dead. I will climb in my hole."

In the depths of the winter the school held an annual cross-country run. I changed into my shorts and shirt and rugby boots and followed the boys and the teachers past the school gates and down the street to a park called the Common, so called because it was designated public land in the thirteenth century. The path went through the gate of the Common, past the lichen-encrusted gravestones of young men who had died in the wars and whole families who had drowned on the *Titanic*, and onward to the big tree by the pond that served as the start line.

I could feel the pain in my chest get worse, and the thought of wanting to stop became so insistent it took all my focus to ignore it and keep my feet hammering the ground. I followed a path that wound through the hedges and brambles deep in the woods. Entering the wood, I came to a narrow trail down which boys lurched single file through knee-deep mud so thick and sticky it swallowed a boot from my foot, stopping me in my tracks to kneel and dig for it. I continued to follow the route through the dense trees. Parts of the trail were overgrown with thorny bushes that formed a corridor of foliage through which I ran as if into a separate world, a wild and primal place of brambles and wet, brown leaves. My legs got scratched and bloody against the thorns. There was no way of knowing how much farther I had to go. I felt my cheeks flush with heat and the sting of the bloody scratches.

Branches and thorny bushes hung low over parts of the trail. Like the telephone box that transported Doctor Who in his journeys through space and time, the woods were larger on the inside than the outside. All I could see ahead of me was a few feet of muddy trail and overgrown plants. I knew I had been here before, in the woods on the Common, though the details of the route in my prior two annual cross-country runs had altogether faded from my mind. After a long time in the thicket, the path would lead out of the woods and back onto the open grass, where I would see the big tree by the pond again. But that was far off in the future. Now all that existed were the brambles slashing my legs and the fear of slowing down and falling back into the mass of boys that huffed behind me.

Rain lashed my face and soaked me to the skin, and soon I was freezing cold and cursing a helpless God who failed to shelter me from the stormy blasts. What this ritual of sadism and soggy stumbling through the mud accomplished I did not know. How pointless everything seemed. Before long I knew that I would finish the loop in the woods and return to the pavilion for a compulsory shower. Mr. Martin, the assistant PE master, would be standing on guard. He used to be in the army. He would stand there, watching, until every last one of us had stripped off our sodden kit and tiptoed shivering underneath the lukewarm water. I would have to stand there among the taller boys with their chest hair and muscles and manly organs, my tiny growth of fledgling pubes and puny chicken legs visible for everyone to see. Then the cross-country run would be over for the year. But then I would face more ordeals. I would finish the third form and then the fourth and fifth form and then the sixth form and then go to university and then get a job like Dad and go to an office every day until I got old and died, following the path into the dismal prison of adult life that our parents and teachers had laid out in front of us, a mindless rush along the course of human existence, which, like the route from the big tree into the cold dark of the woods, I hadn't chosen myself and so wasn't enjoying at all.

But then the path at last led out of the woods, and I could see the big tree by the pond, and I was no longer aware of the cold. I could feel the bloody scratches on my filthy legs and my sodden clothes sticking to my skin and the hard wind blowing in my face and the splashing sound of my rugby boots in the mire and the rhythm of my breathing and moving, no longer urgent and painful but now steady and sustained, as I plodded through the muck and brambles somewhere in the line of boys, some in front and others behind, but feeling indifferent now to where I stood in relation to them, caring only that I was moving and breathing and alive.

Love

The trail leads down to the lake. I follow the course markers along the street to the Tahoe City aid station. I say, "108," announcing my bib number to a race official with a clipboard marking down the runners entering the aid station. No sign of Miriam or the kids. No worries. I'll see them soon, for sure. "There's a guy about a mile back with a broken rib," I tell the official, and give her the runner's bib number. "And another guy maybe five miles back was really frying in the heat. He's moving, but he's going to need some taking care of when he gets here. They both are."

I grab the canvas bag with "108" written on it in black Sharpie pen, which the race organizers have ferried from Homewood along with a pile of similar assorted sacks and totes laid out in a neat rectangular array in numeric order on a tarp next to the food table. Drop bags, they're called. You put bits of kit in them that you don't want to carry with you the whole way but need at certain times, like a jacket and a headlamp for the night. In each bag I've packed socks, shoes, spare clothes, a little first-aid kit for blisters, spare contact lenses, contact lens solution, a toothbrush, and a miniature tube of toothpaste. I've also packed a huge quantity of identical lemon energy bars. When I think of the massive distance still ahead of me, all that seems assured is a certain amount of chaos. To cope with chaos, I have learned to seek comfort in anything constant. I lean my trekking poles against one of the camping chairs beside the table and push my drop bag under the chair. I pick up a paper plate from the end of the table and load it with food, fill a big plastic cup with ice and ginger ale, and sit down. Leaning back in the chair with the canvas material supporting me, I feel an instant relief in my sacrum and the whole way up my spine, the relaxation of all the core muscles after their hard day's labor keeping me upright, marching up thousands of feet and then flying back down the mountain, a radiant sensation of relaxing and opening so lovely it makes me wonder who invented this amazing gizmo, the chair.

I take a slurp of iced ginger ale and then chow down. I've been running for nine hours. I must have burned thousands of calories, and I've covered just 30 miles; 175 to go. In ultras, an upside-down set of rules comes into play: the trail is Wonderland and you are Alice, learning to do the opposite of whatever it makes sense to do in reality. Gluttony is good—a requirement, even. As I heard one wag once observe, all things being equal, an ultramarathon is essentially an eating contest. Over thirty or forty or ninety hours of running, the body burns way more fuel than you could possibly ingest, so it becomes imperative to be as piggy as possible to make up for an energy deficit that widens by the mile and the hour. If there was an ultrarunning rule book, instruction number one would say: "Stuff your face at every opportunity." My plate contains a quesadilla, some salty boiled potatoes and a smattering of chips, peanut-butter-and-jelly sandwiches cut in these darling quarters, piled on with watermelon chunks, mini pretzels, a scattering of chocolate candies, and just a soupçon of pickled gherkin, all washed down with a pint of soda—a fine pairing, I must say. Compliments to the chef. Consider launching your own show: *Salt, Fat, Oreos, Soda*, perhaps. What my dinner lacks in culinary elegance it gains in caloric abundance and in containing enough salt, sugar, starch, and fat in a single meal to induce a coronary in a sedentary citizen but which will sustain my body's chemical needs during my next unknowably long slog of mountain marching until I can chow down again.

A loud belch erupts from all the fizzy drink in my belly. "Excuse me," I say. No one notices or even seems to care. I open my drop bag. I take out a clean pair of socks and a fresh pair of shoes. You wouldn't believe how drenched and filthy shoes get after a day on a mountain trail. Your feet have been stuck in there for hours, cramped and sweaty, as you pound them tens of thousands of times on the dusty, rocky ground. You can do your best to keep all the little bits of grit and twigs and sand from getting in: tie your laces snug, cover your shoes with gaiters. But beyond a certain point you're fighting the basic laws of physics. You can build barriers against nature for a little while, but in the end the dirt gets in. The outside becomes inside.

I clean my feet, put on my fresh socks and shoes and a fresh shirt, then stash the dirty socks, shoes, and shirt in my bag. The old shirt is drenched in sweat and smeared with sunscreen mixed with dirt. I fill both my water bottles, take some candies in a little plastic bag to munch on the trail. I touch my toes to stretch out the backs of my legs and circle my hips to loosen them up. I'm just about ready to leave when my dog, Mochi, comes bounding toward me and leaps up to lick my face. A couple of feet behind Mochi there's Miriam, and my son and daughter, big smiles on all their faces. We hug. Now that Miriam and our kids are here, along with all the junk food and soda, I'm full to the brim with love. Soaking up that much love, I could run forever. I kiss everyone goodbye and run down the trail. Ahead of me I face a two-thousand-foot slog back up a mountain. Make good time and I'll see the view from the high country at sunset.

IV

Earth

The Mourner

It's around six in the evening. The sun's going down. The faraway mountains are bathed in a golden light. The air feels cool. I am listening to a runner tell me how and why she started running. I have no idea how we got into this conversation. On the trail there's this way you just *fall* into random chats with people you've only just met but end up having the deepest conversations of your whole life with. You're in the waking dreamworld, the high country of the mind, everything flowing on the inside and the outside, when along comes another dreamer, and two dreams turn into one. What started off with some comment about the view or our favored brand of trail shoe sent us down a path that's spiraled into our deepest wounds and grief. It must be something about the way everything is moving. You float down the trail. You know where you're going—straight ahead—so there's nothing much you need to think about. It frees up a lot of space for your mind to wander. There's this feeling of your thoughts flowing from one place to the next, and just letting them take you places. Then you end up next to someone else, likely feeling pretty much the same way, and as your feet match each other step for step, your two minds start running together, like intersecting trails.

It reminds me of how Sigmund Freud described free association, only instead of lying down on a couch, observing your thoughts pass by like "a traveler sitting next to the window of a railway carriage,"[10] on the trail you get a nicer view than some old psychoanalyst's office ceiling. The view is not merely interior. You see day change to night and a forest trail leading back up to the high country, and you find yourself remembering another kind of nighttime. "Everyone was dying," she says. "First my best friend dies in a climbing accident. Then it turns out my dad has cancer. There was just this horrible feeling I started to have that death was around every corner. I guess I must've run a bit before in college or whatever. But something took me out to the trail. It felt so *good*. Even when it was bad, it was good. I heard this runner on a podcast once saying there are two types of fun. Type-one fun is sex and ice cream: you like it when it's happening. Type-two fun you like *looking back* on. It's the feeling of mile eighty-six, raining cats and dogs, and you're soaked and freezing and giving God the middle finger, stumbling up some endless hill in the dark with bloody urine and chafing in your asshole, and being back at work five days later, thinking, *That was awesome!* All the bad patches fade away, and all you can remember is the blissed-out bits at the start and what a relief it was to finish and how even the parts that sucked in the middle didn't really suck because it was getting through them that let you know in your bones at the end that you'd really *done something*. And so pretty soon I was hooked. I *had* to run. It was either that or totally fall apart. Every day just *sucked*. But I knew I had this one thing in my life that didn't suck. Running."

"I know what you mean," I say.

"I ran a marathon," says the Mourner. "Then a fifty-miler. Then I went to the wilderness and ran seventy miles solo. When I got back to civilization, I had this incredible feeling. It's hard to put into words . . . I guess the word that comes to mind is *safe*—I felt incredibly safe. I don't just mean in the physical way. That was a part of it, sure. Knowing I was back in the city, safe from the lions and bears. But there was this emotional part too. Like there was nothing to fear. Really, nothing at all. Not even death. I thought, *Everything's okay, just as it is.*"

The sun goes down. I say goodbye to the Mourner and hike onward through the trees. It all feels so familiar, this dark place. Not just in the literal sense that I must have spent hundreds of hours on mountain trails just like this one, slogging uphill in the night, seeing a turn up ahead and marching toward it and then reaching it and making the turn and then seeing more trees, and the next turn, and on and on like that, for what feels like infinity. In the light, back at the start, when your legs are fresh and you're up in the high country and you can see massive distances in every direction, the minutes and steps fly by. You can clock ten miles before you even think to check your watch. But in the night, on tired legs, your view shrinks to a little circle of pale light from your headlamp on the ground and the start of the trees beyond the circle's periphery, and the time compression of the early hours starts to reverse itself. The dark hours drag on and on. I know this feeling well. The trick is to abandon any attachment to getting anywhere and just put your head down and march up the mountain, grunting. *Ugh, ugh, ugh*, I go, trudging uphill in the dark.

..

The parishioners shuffled toward the firepit in the parking lot outside the church, bathed in the flickering orange light, as the priest began chanting the Latin prayers. I gazed into the flames and at the familiar church faces illuminated by their glow. The priest sang in a high monotone, modulating the end of each line upward. The congregation said, "Amen," and then the priest began another prayer. Smoke drifted across the congregation. The prayers ended, and the priest turned from the fire. The altar boys formed a line and proceeded into the church, the flames of the candles carried by the acolytes radiating globes of yellow light, illuminating the aisle ahead. The procession moved in stages. After each movement, the priest said another line of the prayer until we reached the altar, where the procession halted at a row of candles. The congregation gathered closer to the priest. The prayers ended, and the priest began to speak in English, thanking us for braving the cold outside, his voice hushed and gentle. Everyone looked at the burning candles, as if the priest's hush implied a visitation among us, as if the very act of listening implied a sound. Dense clouds of incense floated across the church, dispersing through the congregation, shrouding them in bittersweet unguent, making children cough.

Soon our house smelled of pine needles and brandy and the tree spangled with pink and turquoise fairy lights; perhaps it would snow that year; somewhere there were presents to be found. Sebastian's favorite book was *All About the Bullerby Children* by Astrid Lindgren. It was the only book he read. Was it fourteen times now, or fifteen? "Why don't you read something else?" asked Mummy, but Sebastian didn't want to read anything else. He only wanted to read the adventures of Lars and Pip and Lisa running about in Sweden. "I don't know when Christmas starts in other places, but in Bullerby it starts the day we bake ginger snaps . . ." In Bullerby, it always snowed at Christmas, and I couldn't think of Christmas without thinking of that imaginary snow, suffusing the sodden hills of Hampshire with our winter wonderland of make-believe, for in my mind we were happy Swedish children, no less than Lars and Pip, exploring the hills above Bullerby, a perfect wilderness in which there was not a tree, not a corner of the land, unblanketed by the still-falling snow, unburied by soft white curves and curls, where in the evening the winter sun emerged, like a benediction, to bathe the glacial city in auroras of gold and crimson. Some say magic is real and others that it's a consequence of the human capacity to invest the universe of things with an aura of the numinous. For Sebastian and me at Christmas, the truth lay in between, as matter and mind comingled and our house turned into Bullerby.

··

It's odd to think that I'll likely remember almost nothing of this time. Perhaps this tree over here is the one that memory will preserve. Perhaps that tree over there. Perhaps every remembered tree merges into a single one in the forest of the mind. What feels infinite in the present shrinks in recollection to a couple of snapshots.

I feel great right now, running solo in the dark forest. It's just me and the trees and the trail as they show up in the little white circle of light in front of me from my headlamp. Sometimes I like to stop, turn off my headlamp, and see what real darkness feels like. Miles and miles from civilization, deep under the tree canopy, it is *dark*—a pitch-black vast round shadow that wraps around my eyes like a raven's wings. But even with nothing at all to see, the darkness feels like *something*. A presence, not an absence—or perhaps the presence of an absence. It is quiet, not silent. I feel solitude, not loneliness. Standing very still, I can hear the owls hoot, the flutter of bat wings, the rustle of all the little unseen night creatures as they scurry through the undergrowth. They've been waiting all day for the sun to disappear. And now it's their time, these dark hours when the creatures come flapping and crawling and running through the trees, through the soundless safety of the forest in the night.

The Island of the Cyclops

I gazed through my bedroom window for a long time, wondering what was wrong with me. *Is this normal? Do all fifteen-year-old boys feel like this?* The sensation resembled boredom but hurt in a way that felt like a physical ailment. All the soul was draining out of me. Nothing meant anything; nothing was worth doing. I drifted into an unfamiliar state of consciousness that seemed to stop all thought and freeze my body motionless. Time passed, and for a while this waking dream anesthetized my worry. But the relief was soon succeeded by my recognition of malfunction, an awareness of the frozen state as a kind of trapdoor in the mind into which I had fallen and out of which I might never return. The imperative to escape this paralysis struck me with a surge of anxiety. I jerked my head back and forth, like a dog shaking rain off its fur, and felt my mind restored to vigilance.

I ran through a list of things I could do. My mind went around in circles. Read a book. Write in my diary. Go downstairs and play on the Atari. Go kick a ball in the garden. I could watch television. But it was Sunday afternoon, the beginning of the scheduling wilderness that began with the morning church programs and did not end until *Bonanza*. At the start of the vacation, bad TV was bliss. Waking up the first Saturday after the end of term, going downstairs, and turning on the idiot box, knowing I could stay there the entire day, I felt like Moses reaching the Promised Land. I would sit on the couch next to Sebastian, eating bowl after bowl of chocolate breakfast cereal, watching whatever was on, the stupider the better. In the morning was *Richard and Judy*. They were married in real life, and it was obvious they actually liked each other. You could see it in their eyes, how they smiled and looked at each other and had these little jokes between them. It didn't matter to me what they were talking about.

It could be any random silly thing, like, *Hello! Today we have a man from Preston who makes pancakes*, or, *Now it's time for the weather. Over to you, Simon*. It could really be anything. The point wasn't what they said but how they said it, the way both of them looked right at the camera and through the screen so I was with them, could feel their kind eyes watching me. I didn't know if they had kids. I thought they probably did. One time I wondered what it must be like to be that boy or girl and imagined calling them my mum and dad, and then I imagined any of the boys at school knowing I was thinking something so babyish and I made myself stop imagining it. Richard and Judy were on till about noon. In the afternoon there was *A Country Practice*, and then from four till six there were children's programs, like *Bagpuss* and *The Clangers* and *Grange Hill* and *The Magic Roundabout*, and then the *Six O'Clock News* with Martin Sixsmith, and then after supper there were all the brilliant American shows, like *Dallas* and *Dynasty*, and if I got lucky sometimes a film. Coming up on midnight things got pretty desperate. Sometimes there was something weird and random on, like sumo wrestling, but in the end, around two in the morning, all the programs on all four channels stopped and the screen turned into this multicolored circle with a high-pitched electronic beep . . . If I heard that sound, there really was nothing left to be done except go upstairs and close my eyes and wait till the nature documentaries came on at six. So, yes, I could go downstairs and watch something stupid. But I'd seen enough stupid things downstairs to last a lifetime. It didn't feel good anymore. It had gotten to a point where it felt like my eighth or ninth Easter egg when I was little, or my fourth or fifth pint of my friend Sam's dad's home brew after school that day when I was lying on Sam's bed laughing and listening to New Order and telling him how I felt like I was entering the fifth dimension, but then I puked all over his carpet and tried to stand and go down the stairs, but I was so drunk it was hard to walk, and as I made for the front door so I could get to the station and take the train home, his mum saw me and she said, "Young man, your mother is on her way to pick you up," and I said, "Oh, please don't call my mum, Mrs. McCarthy. Really, I'm begging you. Please."

Then I remembered that Sam had once told me how he went jogging at the weekend. *Run for fun? Run when you didn't have to? What a bizarre idea*, I thought. But jogging was totally different from cross-country or track, said Sam. It was hard to start out with, but it soon got much easier, and there were no teachers yelling at you, and you could go as slow or fast or short or far as you wanted, and once you got into it, there was this amazing feeling. It didn't hurt anymore, and you felt like you could just go and go forever. Really it was the best feeling, said Sam. The feeling of running. And afterward it didn't go away. You could go on feeling that amazing way for hours. You'd be back home doing something boring, but it was like part of you was still on the trail in the woods, winding in and out of the trees. And it was always there. All you needed was your tracksuit and trainers and off you could go again, whenever you wanted.

I put on my tracksuit and trainers and left the house. If I went right, I'd follow our road past the church and my old primary school to the corner shop and the main road that went downhill past the hospital where I was born and the prison and through the pedestrian precinct toward the shops and the church. If I went left, I'd reach the stairs to the underpass to the road on the other side and beyond that I had no idea. I went left.

The whole business felt wrong and weird, an awkward, sweaty, breathless thrash of limbs I was happy no one was there to see and laugh at. After about a hundred yards I was breathing hard and fast and my chest hurt and all I could think about was wanting to stop, but I remembered what Sam had told me about how the hurt would go away, and I kept on going until I reached the end of our road and went down through the underpass, past the woods near the bakery, and down the hill toward the fields at the edge of town. By the time I'd descended the steps to the underpass and walked back up the other side, my breathing had slowed, and the chest pain had subsided with it, so I kept on running.

I realized that I didn't know where I was going. I wasn't lost in the normal sense of the word. The road led in a single direction through a quiet suburban neighborhood I'd seen through car windows countless times and whose corner shops and side roads formed recognizable land-marks that oriented me unambiguously in relation to the way back home. But I felt something novel and disorienting in the experience of being outside by myself, farther from home than I'd ever traveled before on foot, liberated of any practical purpose beyond the basic act of forward motion, a sort of loss that gave me something, the restoration of something unknown yet fundamental, a need each forward footstep started filling even if it didn't yet have a name. As I ran down the road, I became a two-legged sweating animal that nobody was watching. A moving body. A feeling and seeing body. A consciousness formed by the sweaty, breathless effort through the lanes and fields, sensing the birdsong and musty wood smell and crimson evening light converging into one. The road took me to a fence beyond which fields stretched for miles through the countryside. I kept on running as the winter sun sank toward the horizon and the trees shone golden and all my pain melted away and it wasn't until I looked at my watch that I realized that hours had gone by.

ON A SEPTEMBER EVENING a few months before that afternoon I discovered jogging, I went to my bedroom and tried to think about the past. My English teacher had told us to write a story entitled "A Child-hood Memory." My mind went blank. I couldn't remember a single thing that had happened before I was about eleven. The only images that came to mind were from a dream I had once had. It felt like I must have had the dream a very long time ago, when I was little. *I'll write about the memory of a childhood dream.*

I wrote my title, "A Childhood Memory," in neat black curly ink in the middle of the line. I wrote the lowercase initials "hw," short for *home-work*, in the left-hand margin. I wrote the date in numerical form, with the day first and then the month and year, on the right side of the page. I underlined everything with my little plastic ruler. The tails of the letter *h* in *Childhood* and the *m* and *y* in *memory* curled below the line. I made sure when I underlined the title to leave gaps for where the tails dropped below the line, instead of cutting through them.

I remembered the dream: I am on a steam train moving through the countryside. I am sitting in a carriage with all these old ladies and gentlemen. It feels like something from a different century, the days of Queen Victoria maybe. I look at one of the old ladies. Her face has turned into a skeleton. Now I'm not in the train carriage anymore. I'm walking down a cobblestoned street. There are these wrinkled old women fighting over rags—no, bandages. The scene shifts again. Now I'm somewhere else, a junk store, surrounded by old furniture, covered in cobwebs. There's this hat stand I'm looking at. I feel scared. I run away. I can feel the hat stand chasing me, but somehow I know that the hat stand is also the old woman with the skeleton face. I try to run faster, but it feels like I'm stuck. I keep kicking my legs against the ground, but I can't move any faster, like I'm held in place by some invisible force field.

"Intense . . . elliptical, almost impenetrable," wrote my English teacher, Mr. Keene, at the bottom of the page, giving me thirty-three marks out of fifty. For the purpose of my public exams, he said, I would need to write "simpler stories." *How nice that sounds*, I thought. *A simple story*. I knew what he meant. But there was nothing simple about the story I needed to tell.

YES, I THOUGHT, RUNNING farther down the lane, through the fields, everything started going wrong around the time I wrote about that dream. It was hard after that to remember what order things happened in. Events seemed to blur together in my memory. I could remember singing. I could remember screaming. I knew they had happened around the same time. But they felt like two separate worlds.

Some nights later I found myself drunk and scared. At the Bonfire Night party earlier, I had gone upstairs with another boy. We drank a pint of brandy. We took turns, slurping the liquor until we had emptied the pint. I was almost too drunk to stand. I went downstairs. I saw Mum talking to a lady I could remember she had once worked for, the headmistress of a school. I went up to them and said hello. I could see the look of anger on Mum's face. The next thing I knew, I was sitting in the dining room.

I was aware of her yelling and ranting and cursing. I was aware of the feeling inside of being hated. I understood from her torrent of rage that I disgusted her. "You've lost your promise, really gone downhill lost your charms sure you have wee fella you're really rather stupid yes you're mean and stupid you used to be quite clever your headmaster said you were really quite clever when you were younger you were rather nice you were an altar boy played in the garden won the eighty-meter flat race the poetry prize but now you're really very stupid lost your promise really gone downhill lost your charms sure you have wee fella no I can say that yes I can say that I can say whatever the bloody hell I'm a teacher not a typist and you cannot stop me not you I'm not a typist a teacher I used to type one hundred eighty words per minute no you shut up how dare you say that to your mother go to your room this is my house not your house my house not your house why don't you be quiet why don't you keep your mean thoughts to yourself I'm not really interested it's really very boring keep your trap shut keep your gob shut trap shut gob shut you used to be such a nice boy now you're so rude and boring you've really gone downhill lost your charms really very stupid and boring yes I am your mother no you shut up no you shut up no you listen no you shut up shutupshutupshutup—"

I sat in my chair as her rage poured out of her and slammed into me with an avalanching force. I felt utterly helpless, utterly abandoned, powerless to say or do anything at all but sit and withstand the storm of bile and fury until she decided to stop, or unless I could somehow think of the words that might break whatever evil spell had befallen her, to help her remember something. *Mum*, I wanted to say. *I'm your son. Don't you remember your little boy? I know I'm older and bigger now. Some days I'm rude and surly. That's what teenagers are like, sometimes. But I'm still your son. Your child. A human being.* But in my drunken and overwhelmed state those words were not available to me. I sat there sobbing, hoping she might stop, but she kept on raging, and all I could think of to say was "You don't understand that I . . . am good."

Time passed. I have no idea how long. It might as well have been infinity, as if a doorway had opened to a separate dimension of reality, outside time, so that when I recalled that night years after the fact, the memory felt split off from anything before or after, and sometimes I was still there, a helpless boy in a room, feeling hated. At last she did stop yelling and went to make me a cup of strong black coffee, thinking it might sober me up. She didn't put in any milk or sugar. I winced with every mouthful. "Finish it," she said. I complied with her instruction. Another eternity passed. My father entered the room. He sat down next to me. "I know it seems like she's angry with you," he said, "but that's not anger—it's love. She loves you." *Love? Are you an idiot, Dad? Or losing your mind? If that's love, then love must be the most horrible feeling in the world.* I clenched my fists so hard underneath the table that my knuckles went white.

··

A month later I stood in the shadows offstage, in my cowboy boots and ten-gallon hat and gaudy stage mascara—as Curly McLain in the school winter production of the Rodgers and Hammerstein musical *Oklahoma!*—while the school orchestra finished the overture. Feeling enclosed within absolute concentration, I thought of the first word of the opening number. I listened to the flutes and violins. I looked at the wooden house on the stage. I took deep breaths to calm myself. Memories of my disgrace on Bonfire Night had vanished to a separate domain of my consciousness, the shadow land of crying and feeling helpless and hated. The orchestra fell silent. *"There's a bright golden haze on the meadow,"* I sang. *"The corn is as high as an elephant's eye, and it looks like it's climbing clear up to the sky."* As I walked onstage, the orchestra launched into the lovely melody of the musical's opening number, "Oh, What a Beautiful Mornin'." Illuminated by searing yellow stage lights, the little wooden imitation farmhouse shone with an almost cartoon luminosity. The school assembly hall was full of people, all the way to the back and on every row in the balcony, a crowd of hundreds. I felt the power of our voices, and of a feeling of immersion in an alternate world that had taken, it seemed, half the school to make—the actors and cellists and oboists, the boys who had built the set and made the lights work, the teachers who had taught us to sing and act and had helped us with our costumes, all the friends and family members who had come to watch and clap and sing along. But then I felt a wrenching sadness, as if shaken awake from a magical dream, when I walked into school on the day after the show's last night, and tried to cope with the thought I would never be happy again.

In the following six months, my focus drifted from schoolwork. In the early summer of 1985, I sat my first two public exams, known in England as O Levels. I entered the exam hall. I took my seat. Midway through the math exam, the paralyzed feeling came over me. I sat there, frozen, unable to think. After the English exam, I swapped notes with Perry, a boy I sometimes sat with on the train to school. He asked me about one of the comprehension exercises in the exam. It referred to a passage about a person reacting in a certain way "for fear the house might fall." What might the author be attempting to convey through this image of a falling house? "It's obviously a metaphor for the collapse of something larger, right?" said Perry. "I said the British Empire—the rest of the poem was about the colonies. What did you put?" I remembered that in the stress of the exam the figurative meaning had been completely lost on me. I had taken the sentence at face value and said so on my answer sheet. But Perry was right, it was obvious. I didn't tell him. I felt afraid.

AMERICA! THE VERY WORD sounded like a marching band. Look, here comes Mickey Mouse and Obi-Wan, here comes Spider-Man and

Van Halen singing "Jump"; here comes Curly and Laurey riding in the surrey with the fringe on top, beneath the Rocky Mountains, exactly like they looked on Dad's Coors T-shirt; here comes Marty McFly in rocket shoes and the boundless frontier of the future world. We'd landed in JFK at night and took a cab into Manhattan. Colossal illuminated towers came into view, magisterial and holy, like concrete hands held aloft to Creation: What minds had made such marvels? We stayed in a bed-and-breakfast in an apartment hundreds of feet from the ground. I was kept awake by car horns and police sirens and people whistling and yelling. We explored Manhattan. I followed my mother and father into a SoHo bookstore. I looked at the expensive hardback art books displayed in the center of the store. As I was leaving, I made eye contact with the store owner. He smiled at me. "We're going now," my mother said. The store owner gave me a small paperback book, the contents of which I didn't have time to register. "I wouldn't want you to have to leave here empty-handed," he said, laughing, the enigmatic cadence of his sentence prompting a conspiratorial look that flashed between the store owner and his grinning young male assistant. We got into a taxi. An atmosphere of menace pervaded the cab's interior. "Do you understand what those American fellas were doing?" my mother said. "Yes," I lied. "They were homosexuals. Men who have sex with each other. Are you a homosexual?" "No," I said. I shuddered with dark rage. *Who the hell are you to tell me who I can talk to? I'm not gay. At least I don't think so—not that it should matter. And straight or gay, my sexuality is none of your fucking business.* I started to cry. "I hope you don't get AIDS," she said.

From Kennedy Airport we flew to Los Angeles, where we saw the pits of tar into which mammoths and saber-toothed tigers had fallen in the Paleolithic era and where after a chilly dip in the Pacific I ordered a waffle piled six inches high with whipped cream and blueberries—it was the most expensive item on the menu and my father complained that we couldn't afford it. "Why do you always have to ruin everything?" my mother said to my father. "Sorry," he said. The waffles arrived—a huge stack of which I could only manage half. Our next stop was Vegas. A teenage girl emerged from the giant hotel pool, jewels of water sparkling in the summer desert sunlight on her lean, tan body. I had seen her chatting to a muscular Frenchman in the shallow end, how she laughed at his jokes and said, *"Oui, d'accord,"* in a twang like a *Dynasty* character. I watched her walk to one of the white plastic pool recliners and put on mirror shades and lie down.

"À bientôt, Jacques," she said, winking, as the Frenchman left the pool and waved goodbye. The girl lay motionless as the jewels of water evaporated from her skin in the oven-like Nevada heat. She sat upright and lathered her body with sunblock and then reclined again, aquamarine ripples from the pool reflecting in her shades.

Knowing Mum and Dad, our itinerary was a mystery. Even the next hour might well entail a lurch into chaos. I had to make my move that very second. I remembered something Sam had told me. Sam had been on holiday in the US the previous summer. "Yank girls go mad for English accents," he said. Open your mouth uttering English-sounding words and a gorgeous American girl would stick her tongue in there right away. I went up to the girl and sat down next to her. "Hello," I said. Silence. "I am from England," I said. Silence. I could think of nothing else to say, so I leapt into the pool and swam the crawl until my triceps started cramping. Then I got out of the pool and lay down and looked at my paper-white skin and realized there was no hope whatsoever of going back to England with a suntan, and then I followed Mum and Dad inside for lunch. The buffet was all-you-can-eat, a goal whose outer limits I was reluctant to explore: a day or so before I'd watched Sebastian at a casino eatery, likewise licentious of gluttony, load his dinner plate high with shark, lobster, beef, shrimp, pasta, turkey, and mashed potatoes—more-than-he-could-eat, it turned out—and flee from the restaurant to throw it all up in the toilet.

After lunch we got back into the car, and from Vegas we drove to Arizona. I stared at the dry wilderness that stretched in sci-fi technicolor hues to arid crags in every direction. The highway extended to a far-away mountain pass, beyond which extended expanse upon expanse of scorched dust and emptiness. I don't remember where we stopped when my father tired of driving—conceivably it was Flagstaff. The next day, or the one after—that time is a desert in my memory—I stood at the South Rim of the Grand Canyon and looked down, contemplating an immensity of such scale it swallowed up all prior notions about what big was supposed to look like. The North Rim was so distant it had different weather, clouds in fortresslike formations that stacked through the day and erupted in forks of lightning.

I endured more time in the car. One morning we left a motel in a hurry—who knows why. We were hundreds of miles away, possibly no longer in Arizona, when my mother opened her suitcase and couldn't find all her clothes. I'd seen her put some of them in one of the drawers near the television in the previous night's motel. I kept this recollection to myself; if I told Mum I knew where she'd put her clothes, I'd be the one who took all the blame.

"Somebody must have stolen them!" she said.

"I don't think so," my father said.

"It was that Navajo woman who came into our room. The cleaning lady. The Navajo stole my clothes."

Sometime later I was eating clam chowder from a bread bowl on a foggy late afternoon at a restaurant on the wharf at San Francisco Bay when the conversation turned to anticipation of the next school year and the arrival in about a week of my exam results. I stared into the distance and felt my mind go blank.

About a week later, back home, I was lying in bed one morning when I heard the mail flop onto the doormat downstairs. My heart beat faster with dread. I got out of bed. I left my room. I went across the landing. I reached the staircase. I walked downstairs. I wished I could leap into the next millennium or turn into a dog in France—be anything except me there and then, a fifteen-year-old boy about to learn the results of my first two public exams. I saw that a skinny envelope sat upon the doormat. I saw my name written on the envelope in small black capital letters, and in the top left-hand corner I saw the words

OXFORD AND CAMBRIDGE EXAMINATION SCHOOLS. I walked back to my room with the letter. I sat on the edge of my bed. My mother followed me into the room and sat down next to me. I opened the letter. I took out the little slip of white paper inside it. I looked at the words on the paper. A moment passed between my sight of my grades and the catastrophic meaning my mind attached to them, like the pause between a child's fall to the ground and the cry registering his shock.

English Language   B
Mathematics   C

What a disgrace. "Oh no," I said. "Well, that's just terrible, isn't it?" said my mother. I detected in her tone a feeling toward me of utter disgust and contempt. I might as well have heard a judge's verdict for a heinous crime. A wave of shame engulfed me. I burst into tears. My mother left me alone in my room, weeping.

I cried for hours. I cried until my eyes stopped making tears. I kept remembering my mother's scornful words. I wished that I could forget them. But the memory of her voice of hatred refused to fade away, and the sting of shame that this memory induced in me only seemed to build upon itself with each unbidden recollection, as if her remembered voice had formed a kind of indelible footnote in the margins of my awareness,[*] forcing my mind forever to run back and forth between the reality of the present moment and the recurring insult that resounded in the background of consciousness. It was the loudest sound in the world, but I alone could hear it.

Sometime later that morning Sebastian walked past me. I saw him examine me with a look of pity and curiosity, as if Mum had instructed him to preserve my isolation. I picked up a paintbrush and began to paint the walls. We'd been redoing the paintwork in the previous week. As I brushed the white paint on the walls, I became aware of the space

---

[*]   *"Well, that's just terrible, terrible, terrible, terrible . . ."*

inside, where the feeling of Me used to be, collapsing into nothing. *I can't believe how stupid I've been. I don't understand why I ruined everything.*

In the mornings I painted the walls while listening to classical music albums on Dad's hi-fi. I couldn't imagine the words of any human language adequately describing my perception of self-implosion, the impression that in place of the phenomenon where the pronoun *I* formerly stood as a signifier an anguished abyss had broken open. The only music I could tolerate was equally wordless. Among the stack of Dad's albums on the living room shelves I found a record by the composer Penderecki called *Utrenja: The Entombment of Christ.* I heard voices droning and muttering and wailing in a language I didn't know and screeches and cries in a cavernous silence as within this cacophony I received a communication: *Others have suffered the abyss before me. There are no words for this stab in the soul I am feeling. But there is a sort of music. Someone understood the feeling. Someone felt the horror of the dark and turned it into sound.*

IN THE *PHAEDRUS,* PLATO says that our best explanations of the world are those which classify phenomena according to objective underlying categories, or "carve nature at its joints."

Theories across the centuries have proceeded with that Platonic ambition in mind, from those of nineteenth-century German psychiatrist Emil Kraepelin—who sorted his observations of people regarded as insane into two categories, dementia praecox and manic depression (the diagnoses later known as schizophrenia and bipolar disorder, respectively)—to the current proliferation of 297 mental disorder categories in the fifth edition of the American Psychiatric Association's *Diagnostic and Statistical Manual of Mental Disorders (DSM-5).* Psychiatric labels can be stigmatizing, but they can also be useful: they organize inexpressible chaos into linguistic form. Looking back as a clinician now, I could likely hazard a diagnosis for my mother, my father, and me. But I won't. Even assuming I could be objective, I don't have much data to go on—really just the contents of my own fallible memory. And even in some science-fiction parallel universe where I could travel by time machine back to 1986 and administer a battery of psychological tests to my parents and produce an accurate diagnosis, to convey such information would be to falsify the experience I lived through, the traumatic nature of which was in no small part constituted by the absolute absence of any kind of organizing theory, in my mind or anyone else's, to sort the sad, scary madness of our family's implosion in neat and comprehensible categories, to tell me or Sebastian or Mum or Dad what was happening to us, and what we might do to keep our family from collapsing.

I must have been aware on some level—in the instinctive way children and even dogs and cats can sense the presence of danger—of seismic ruptures in my family life, cascading from the feelings of fear and confusion I had experienced since my early childhood. Years later I would come to trace the sequence of perplexing alterations in my mother's behavior that had begun to manifest about four years earlier. She had an affair and invited my father to embark on a similar liaison. She changed jobs several times, following intense verbal confrontations with colleagues, and then became unemployed. She sent a series of letters to my uncle and aunt containing obscene and threatening language, which prompted my uncle to consider legal action against her. She spent money in a compulsive and reckless manner. Debts accumulated.

My father recalled a period of depression she had suffered years earlier, when I was a small child, for which she had received antidepressant medication, and he understood her subsequent behaviors as symptoms of a mental illness. Yet she presented no signs to him of understanding herself as ill and resisted all attempts to seek the few forms of treatment then available. It occurred to him that in the absence of psychotherapy she might be amenable to family therapy, but this too she declined.

One of the central features of both bipolar disorder and schizophrenia is a phenomenon called anosognosia, an inability of the person suffering an illness to recognize that they are ill. Great skill on behalf of clinicians can be required to engage people with those conditions in any form of treatment, because they do not think of their experiences in terms of illness. My father implored his beloved Clara to seek help—for the sake of their marriage; for the sake of our family's survival; for the sake of her own sanity—but she could not or would not listen. She was impossible. There was nothing more he could do. So he gave up trying.

Years later he told me what had happened to him. His worries had begun when Gran sold the house by the sea in Ireland and moved to England. Though he hadn't lived there since he had left home in his teens, the loss of his childhood home perturbed him with a novel anguish. It seemed to him that he was now forever severed from the past, the land of his Irish ancestors, the green hills and forests and rivers through which he had wandered as a boy. His thoughts drifted to his father, dead for a decade but whose loss he now began to feel with a sense of regret and impossible yearning. "I wasn't sure if I'd ever really talked to him," he told me years later. "Not really, I mean. Obviously we spoke. But we'd never really talked. He was just there, in the background. And I suppose in some childish way I thought he always would be. Then he was gone. But for years I didn't really know he was gone, you know? It sounds silly, but while I could still go back to the house, it felt like he was still there somehow. Like my father was part of the house. But once the house was gone, I really knew he was gone. He was never coming back." His mind then turned to a path not traveled from his childhood days as a mathematics prodigy. He could have become a math professor. He could have spent his days focused on a timeless realm of pure abstraction and infinite possibility. When and why and how did he abandon his boyhood's wonder at the infinite? How had he wound up a middle-aged working stiff, married to this woman, once so lovely, now transforming in such an incomprehensible way?

In the spring of 1986, my mother was admitted to the hospital for a medical procedure, for which she received general anesthesia. As my father stood by the hospital bed after the operation and my mother started to talk, he had the distinct impression, he told me when we began to speak of our family's collapse about a decade later, when I was in my mid-twenties, that she had somehow changed. He could not quite say how. It was as if he were examining a family photograph that had shifted out of focus: a change so subtle that it was hard to identify whether the alteration resided in Clara or in his own vision. The transformation reminded him of a phenomenon he had encountered in Celtic mythology. There are stories in Celtic legend, he told me, of spirits called the sidhe that enter the human world to kidnap souls. To live on Earth, the sidhe require bodies to live in, so they kidnap souls and take them to the faery world so they can use the human body as a host. On Earth, the person still appears to be alive, but everything about their personality has changed. When a person underwent a radical change in their personality, the Celts said that person was "away with the faeries," my father explained. He understood that science offered another kind of explanation, invoking disordered biological mechanisms in the brain, whose objective validity he did not dispute. But the jargon of science fell short of articulating his unbearable feeling of loss. To name the feeling, myth still offered a closer match: Clara was gone. She was away with the faeries.

By the following June, clear differences were observable in my mother's handwriting and signature. Until September 1986, she used her first name and surname. Nine months later, she used her initials and surname, appending both with the acronyms for her undergraduate degree and teaching credential. In the second of the two signatures, she formed the capital letter *C* that begins her forename with the bottom curve of the letter extending below the other letters.

But I knew almost none of this at the time. By the time I understood that a profound transformation had occurred in her, and thus in all of us, many years had passed. Few of the early warning signs of psychological trouble were discernible to my teenage self—she was the only mother I had ever had, and I had nobody to compare her to. When, in my twenties, I started looking back and wondering what had happened, recollecting my experiences of those years, I could remember everything *but* her, as if she were present as an absence. Most of what I could remember were feelings, perceptions of what seemed at the time like axioms of the universe, a sense of dread or fear or hopelessness that reflected something basic about the world, something everyone understood but agreed not to talk about. It seems likely to me that she suffered from bipolar disorder with periods of psychosis in the manic phases of her illness. But all I knew at the time was that my mother had gone mad. Nothing was more frightening and tragic than madness. And it was happening to my family. My parents had gone mad—maybe all of us had. I felt ashamed. I seldom spoke about my family or the confusing parts of my own mind to others, even close friends, and focused my energy on putting as much distance as I could between the functional human I impersonated in public and the madman I feared I might be.

EACH DAY THAT SUMMER passed into the next with a feeling of desolation. In the mornings I would walk our Dalmatian, Maeve, around the neighborhood and in the afternoons paint the walls and listen to *Utrenja*, contemplating the ruin of my life, a disaster of my own making. I could remember the Good Boy I used to be, a few years before, until I started drinking. I used to be going somewhere. But not anymore. I had destroyed my future. Day after endless day passed in this desolate state. I had disappeared. There was nothing left of me. Darkness had swallowed me whole. I lacked language to name my feelings. I would have coped better if someone had been there to help me understand what I felt or provide a wider perspective. *It's not the end of the world. You got a couple of so-so grades this time. No big deal. In a couple of weeks you'll be back at school, and you can focus on next year. You have nothing to be ashamed about. Remember that we care about you. These were exams, not a final verdict on your entire life.* But no one said this.

Two weeks passed. One afternoon my mother came into my room. "Would you like me to help you with your English?" she said. "I am a teacher. I can help children with English." "Yes," I said. She sat down next to me. She showed me a book of language comprehension exercises. They had the "See Jane run" feel of questions aimed at much younger children. I went through the exercises, sitting next to Mum. *Where is*

Spot? Spot is chasing Jane. It was little-kid stuff, I knew. But I could do it. *I* could do it. I felt myself coming back from the Darkness. By the time the new school year began the following week, I felt like a different person. *The old me is gone*, I thought. *That silly kid who sat at the back of the class, writing nonsense in my notebook, getting drunk on Sam's dad's home brew: what a fool.* I threw all my diaries into the trash. I sat at the front of the class and stopped talking to Sam. I focused on every single word of every teacher in every single class every day of the week as if my life depended on it. Under no circumstances whatsoever would I tolerate another collapse into the abyss.

A LITTLE WHITE CIRCLE of light from my desk lamp lit up the books in front of me. The world inside the circle of light was pure and clear and logical. I could stay there all night. I had never felt such clarity and focus. When it got past 1 a.m. I would sometimes feel my energy starting to fade. I yearned to go to bed. Then I would glance at the exam results paper from the Oxford and Cambridge Examination Schools, which I had pinned to the corkboard above my desk, and a memory of the day the letter flopped onto the doormat would rush into my mind with a jolt of terror that would shock me back to vigilance.

I had to stay awake. If I stayed vigilant, I could see the path that led ahead of me from Cannon Road to Oxford. Where that path might lead after Oxford, I didn't know. But one thing was certain: by then these days in Cannon Road would have faded into memory. Perhaps I would become a doctor, perhaps a writer. Both seemed like worthwhile occupations. A doctor put broken people back together; a writer served as a witness to our broken world. Though to follow the writer path would surely piss off Mum. She might throw another glass of whiskey at my head, like the time I told her I was thinking about studying literature at university. I understood that reading books had gotten her absolutely nowhere. After all her years in the library, buried in Joyce and Austen, she was unemployed. Better to be a thinker than a dreamer, she said.

You couldn't do both. Either way, I had to stay awake and memorize everything for my exams, even if it meant working into the wee hours.

I memorized the first twenty chemicals in the Periodic Table of Elements as a single word: HHeLiBeBCNOFNeNaMgAlSiPSClArKCa. I memorized Book IX of Homer's *The Odyssey* in ancient Greek. Odysseus, I would be sure to remember, was finding his way home after the great battles described in *The Iliad*. Along the way, he met the one-eyed monster Polyphemus, who captured Odysseus and his men and came close to eating them, until our hero tricked his way out of the situation, enraging his cyclopean foe. "Hear me, great Neptune," yelled Polyphemus. "If I am indeed your own true-begotten son, grant that Odysseus may never reach his home alive."

Everything felt as sharp as crystal. I could read a page of ancient Greek and commit it to memory in minutes. I would stay awake with my studies till the wee hours, then sleep just five or six hours, then go to school, marveling at the clean and perfect feeling that came from solving simultaneous linear and quadratic equations or memorizing the second-person singular future perfect of irregular Greek verbs in the optative or the chemical formula of glycogen. In the evening after supper, as I cleaned and dried the dishes, I would notice how the world seemed to shrink to my awareness of the aluminum sink and the dish drying in my hands and the sink draining as I watched the spiral motion of the water disappear, dried the basin with a paper towel and mopped every last droplet of water on the faucet and polished the basin until it shone like a crystal mirror.

Inside the little circle of white light on my desk, the world made sense. When I woke in the morning and took the train to school, I felt as if the circle of light formed a force field around me, a protective sphere beyond whose frontiers I saw the world with crystalline precision and no emotion. Nothing could hurt me anymore. I had the Eye of the Cyclops.

Yet beyond the perimeter of my cyclopean vision, I understood that unusual events were occurring. Just as I split my awareness off from the possibility of pain, my parents' minds were beginning to fracture and fragment. Put the mind under conditions of great stress and perception shrinks to a tiny sphere. What counts is getting through the danger *now*. Surviving. Evolution has shaped the nervous system to shift gears fast when it senses imminent disaster. Your attention sharpens and narrows. When the house is on fire, you run for the door. Your heart is pumping; your eyes are fixed on the exit. Your conscious attention splits off from the peril pursuing you, shoving unbearable perceptions or feelings aside. In this dissociative state, your awareness collapses to a tiny sphere, enclosing only those facts of perception salient in that very instant to survival. What memory records from such encounters with catastrophe will necessarily comprise a scattering of luminous fragments. Much of the experience as you lived through it at the time then vanishes in the void. The brain doesn't bother to store all those minor details, because a crisis tends to take psychic shape as a sole imperative: Get. The. Hell. Out.

One evening I went downstairs to the kitchen to discover that the pantry shelves were bare. I went to look for my father. I found him in the living room, pacing back and forth, dressed in the same striped business shirt he'd been wearing for several days. "Dad, we need food," I said. His eyes met mine and looked away again as he continued with his walk from one end of the room to the other and back again, twisting a frond of his curly hair with the index finger of his left hand until it wound into a knot. "You need to get in the car and take me to McDonald's," I said. He followed me out of the house. We got in the car. He drove us out our road and followed the road plunging steeply into town. The car picked up speed. "Slow down," I said. His glazed eyes stared dead ahead of him. "Slow down!" I said. The car slammed against the curb. I felt a jolt of panic. I braced myself for disaster. The car lurched back onto the road and slowed down. He parked outside McDonald's. I ordered burgers and fries and milkshakes for Sebastian and me. We drove home in silence.

For some time, I came to understand much later, my father's mind had been drifting into the waking nightmare of a terrifying psychosis. He couldn't sleep. He couldn't think. One night he went into his room to discover that his bed had disappeared. In its place he saw a giant pile of human filth, its surface pulsing and rippling, as if it were wriggling with a million worms. He left the room in a state of terror. Now he understood. He called the parish priest. "I saw the devil," he said. "The end of the world is coming. People must be warned!"

I knew nothing of my father's ghastly hallucination at the time. I saw a worried man in a stinky shirt pacing in the living room. I knew he was unwell. But I utterly lacked the knowledge to understand the nature of his illness or how I was supposed to accommodate my awareness of his suffering other than by ignoring it and keeping my mouth shut. Then one night I was in my room, studying, when I heard the doorbell. Mum opened the door. I heard voices downstairs. I went to the top of the stairs. Our family doctor stood in the hall. He had his brown leather bag in one hand. Dad followed him into the living room. The doctor closed the door. I went to bed. When I went downstairs for breakfast in the morning, Dad was gone. "Your father's in the hospital," said Mum. "He had a nervous breakdown."

Nervous breakdown: it meant he'd gone mad. Madness was the bogeyman that lurked beyond the frontiers of rationality. The English zeitgeist with respect to mental illness had in essence not evolved in any meaningful way since medieval times. In Britain in the 1800s, poor people with mental illness were locked in prison as *pauper lunatics*. By the mid-1980s, mad people in England were no longer assumed by definition to be criminals. But anyone unfortunate to find him- or herself afflicted by an illness of the mind continued to suffer a different sort of incarceration: the prison of silence and shame. "Don't tell anyone," said Mum. "It's a secret."

We went to visit Dad in the hospital the following night. He was sitting on the edge of his bed, fully clothed and clean-shaven, staring dead ahead, his eyes dazed. "Hello, Dad," I said, but he didn't hear me. Didn't seem to know I was even there. When I sat beside Sam in morning assembly at school the following Monday, he asked about my weekend. "My dad went to the hospital," I said. "Oh no. What happened?" said Sam. "He had a nervous breakdown," I said. "Oh . . . God," said Sam, scrunching up his face like he'd caught a whiff of sour milk. *Don't talk about it. Don't even think about it.*

It was a springtime day and the raindrops sparkled in the daffodils when Dad came home from the hospital about a month later. In his bright new sweater, he looked like a little boy dressed up for church on Sunday. "Thanks for taking care of everything while I was gone," he said.

I had imagined that my father's return from the hospital would precipitate the return to a semblance of stability in our home. I was wrong. The shifts in my mother's behavior whose onset I had noticed some years earlier metastasized in a baffling and global transformation of the person I once knew. I couldn't follow what she was talking about. One night I went to her room to tell her I was going into town when she began to speak. She said something like "I need two pounds for a coffee—not half a pound of tuppenny rice. I lost ten pounds with Weight Watchers at King Alfred's College. Arthur pulled Excalibur from the stone. Everybody should get stoned. They stone women to death in Saudi Arabia for adultery. They should stone Dr. Riding. I am Mrs. Thompson, bachelor of arts degree. What about Professor Fisher? Come with me and I will make you fishers of men . . . Nuclear fission—we were with CND at Greenham Common. I once had a notion for a boy in Ireland who was a fisherman. He drowned, of course . . . All of us drown in something, sea or sorrow. I drowned my sorrows in whiskey when your father went away. You learned to swim in California when you were three. Then to the isles of Greece, the four of us, do you remember? I was out of my depth back then. A lovely Swede came rushing to my rescue. Like one of those fellas from ABBA—*'Super Trouper, lights are gonna find me.'* You used to like ABBA, didn't you? ABBA, father . . . *Eli, Eli, lama sabachthani* . . . Into thy hands I commend my spirit. Do not despair. One of the thieves was saved. The Navajo stole my clothes in Arizona, you remember? Monument Valley. Yea, though I walk through the valley of death, rode the six hundred. We rode horses when you were five. Straight from the horse's mouth. All mouth and no trousers . . ."

I tried to understand what she was saying, but the links between the meanings of her words felt random, as if she were following a trail inside her mind that she felt compelled to wander, like a child in a fairy tale lost in a forest of language. I would stand at the foot of her bed, listening, joining her for a while on a trail into a dreamworld through which I could sense her desire for me to follow, detecting her need for me to stay with her inside it, perhaps because she believed we had visited parts of that world together in the past. I would sense, too, her recognition of me as a companion who might find the way in this dreamworld, yet I noticed also that she didn't appear to register my reluctance to do so. I experienced this fracture between us as an isolation I bore alone. But then as I listened, and she continued to speak, I would feel my attention drift away from her, until my mind went blank. I wished she would stop talking, so I could stop listening and leave, but on and on she would travel, meandering through her dreamworld, until I would start to fear that unless I moved my body that very instant, the sound of her droning on, inaudible and unintelligible beyond the horizon of my awareness, would become a kind of hypnotic spell that might freeze me forever where I stood at the end of her bed. So as her words kept running this way and that through the dream forest of her mind, I would say goodbye to her and leave the room.

OUR NEW HOUSE ON Fairgreen Road was much smaller than the house on Cannon Road, a narrow two-story red-brick terrace about halfway down a row of identical buildings near the center of town. An accumulation of debt had forced my father to sell the house I had grown up in, and overnight we lost the physical connection to the solid world of the garden and the Jungle and the life before all the madness. A vast body of other traces of our past vanished in the move, including most of our books and records and photographs. When I asked Dad where all our books had gone, he shrugged and said he didn't know. I might as well have asked him if there could be a connection between the Loch Ness Monster and the Illuminati. All that remained of the books on Cannon Road was *Atlantis*. On the living room wall was a family portrait my mother had commissioned from a professional photographer. Mum sits grinning in the middle with Dad on one side and Sebastian on the other. That's me in the right-hand corner, losing all religion: leather jacket, crimped hair, black circles under my eyes.

Mum kept the electric heater on even on the warmest days. She refused to keep a trash can in the kitchen. She instructed us to dispose of our trash in the plastic bags she hung from a hook on the kitchen wall. The bags would split and strew chicken bones and used plastic microwave lasagna containers all across the floor. When one day I asked my father about the absence of a trash can, he said, "Mum doesn't want one," and that was that.

We spent most nights watching television. Sebastian sat in one chair, me and Dad on the couch. I was conscious of my mother droning on in the background. One night Sebastian told her to be quiet, and she picked up a steel clock from the mantelpiece and tried to smash him in the head. He defended himself with a kung fu block.

The nights of silence punctuated by bizarre rages continued. I couldn't bear it. "Why don't you do something?" I said to my father. "About what?" he said. "About Mum," I said. "Well, why don't you do something?" he said. Outside the house, in public, I felt the anguish of recognizing that my mother's disorientation was conspicuous to other people, conferring shame upon me as the son—I had come to realize—of a madwoman.

Sometime later we went out for dinner in a restaurant on the high street. The waiter came to take our order. "Do you speak French?" my mother said. *Oh Jesus no—please someone make her stop.* "Not really," the waiter said. I could detect the confusion in her voice and eyes. My father sighed, his head downcast. "*Je parle Français. Parlez vous Français? Je suis un rock star*—like Bryan Ferry. Or Van Morrison. The Chieftains—a sense of wonder . . . Didn't I come to bring you—What about German? Do you speak German?" The waiter communicated that she had not studied German. "Sebastian here is excellent at German. He went to the Berlin Wall. *Sprechen Sie Deutsch? Ich bin ein Berliner.* What else, Sebastian? 'Ask not what your country can do for you'—*Eins . . . zwei . . . drei*—" I wanted to be somewhere else. I wanted to be *someone* else. Anywhere and anyone but there, then, being me. A half-smile formed on the waiter's mouth, and she laughed with an expression I recognized as embarrassment. Sebastian and I made eye contact with each other, a sad mutual awareness forming in our gaze, as if the two of us were cast adrift on an island far away, two young residents of a land cut off in the ocean where among the two older inhabitants one was helpless and the other had gone insane.

Life inside the walls of the house felt ever more unreal. I took refuge in the world outside. How strong my legs felt on the road and trail! And what a relief it was to embrace the fire that ignited in my chest and heart and folded me within it, as my legs hammered the ground, and I absorbed the knowledge that the ground communicated of the earth's stable presence underneath me and the solid feeling it gave me inside. With every step forward, the house fell farther behind. And I knew that this solid feeling would always be there for me: all I had to do was put on my running shoes and get outside. I ran to build a foundation for the formless feelings inside me that I didn't understand. I ran to persuade myself that one day I would leave all the madness of my family's past behind and never look back. I ran to remember what was real.

Years passed. I left my family's past behind. But then I did look back. It was hard to remember what was real, or understand why so much of my memory of those days of madness had vanished into oblivion. I wondered about everything that I had forgotten, and everything that was later irrecoverable because I had never truly known it at the time: the world outside my tiny sphere of Cyclopean vision. And so years later, pacing the hospital corridor, trying to recall those lost days in Cannon Road, all I could remember was a white sphere of light, and a boy in a room looking at the book inside it, memorizing what the Cyclops had told Odysseus, in the words of a dead and ancient language.

Hope Is a Hymn

I held a pebble in my palm and wrote down how it felt cold and hard and round. I observed the little Labrador that came to visit from the animal charity. I played the conga drum. I painted a mandala whose outer rim was radiant in pink and orange and whose core was a sphere of darkness. In the evenings, Miriam would come during visiting hours with bags of Chinese takeout. I watched her unwrap the cartons of noodles and sweet-and-sour vegetables, recognizing them as the relics of a ruined ancient civilization that some distant ancestor of mine might have lived in long ago. In group therapy in the morning, I listened to the sad stories from both newcomers and some familiar faces: Holst, the Shopkeeper, the Prisoner, La Llorona.

One day the conversation veered toward the circumstances that had brought us to the hospital. "I took a bunch of pills and liquor," said Holst. "I was okay with being dead. I didn't want it to hurt. I figured, *I'll get high enough that I won't feel anything.* Then I got in the bathtub and I opened up a vein." He gestured at the bandage on his arm.

I won't feel anything: I hid this nugget in a secret chamber of my mind.

Seven days had passed since my arrival in the hospital. I had the measure of the place. *This place is doing nothing for me*, I thought. It troubled me to imagine what I assumed would be lifelong negative consequences for assenting to psychiatric hospitalization.

The social worker on the ward did her best to convince me otherwise. Her name was Sandra. She went by her first name and addressed me likewise. She came to the ward dressed in jeans and a sweatshirt. She invoked the concept of *recovery* and used the phrase "Right on" in every other sentence. I felt much more comfortable talking to her than either Dr. Browning or Dr. Hewitt.

"Soon you'll be out of here and getting back to work," said Sandra.

"But I don't wanna go to work," I said. "I hate it."

"Work in general or what you're doing now?"

"My job right now. I'm a grant writer. I thought it had something to do with writing. It doesn't."

"What else would you like to do?"

"I don't know. There are a million things."

"Right on. Like what?"

"I go round in circles. I can't decide."

"Well, tell me a couple. What do you think you'd like to do?"

"I don't know. I can't do anything. I can listen to other people talk. I used to think maybe I could do something like what you do, counseling whatever, but now I'm not allowed."

"What are you talking about?"

"Because of being a mental patient."

"That doesn't matter. There are laws against discrimination. When you get better, you can do anything you want."

You can do anything. Was it true? In Sandra's presence, I could almost believe in the future again. But the belief disappeared the second Sandra did. My faith in the future was like my teenage faith in God. While I was inside church and saying Hail Marys and joining in an old familiar hymn, I could feel my lips move and the words come out without needing to think about them. There was something nice about the feeling, so familiar and automatic, even if I didn't believe in God or Jesus or heaven anymore. The image of a livable future, which emerged in my mind when a believer like Sandra spoke of it, had the same transient existence. Hope was a hymn. It had a comforting sound. Once Sandra was gone, the future disappeared along with her. When I had told her that one day I might want to listen to people for a living, I wasn't lying. In her presence, it was the truth. But in her absence, nothing was true.

After nine days in the unit, I met one late morning with Sandra and Dr. Browning and Miriam. Dr. Browning told Miriam that I wasn't feeling suicidal anymore because that's what I'd told Dr. Browning.

Sandra said "Right on" at least twice and told Miriam about the out-patient program I would be starting after the weekend. "Just keep an eye on him over the weekend, and if you're worried, give us a call," said Dr. Browning, signing my discharge papers and leading me and Miriam to the door of the ward. The doctor unlocked the door, and I followed Miriam down the hall and took the elevator from the fourth floor down to the lobby and out to the street.

Two days later I stood in the church pews at Glide Memorial, listening to the choir. In my anguished state of mind their voices resembled a wall of noise without meaning or emotion.

I feel nothing here, I thought. *All hope is gone.*

I left the church. I went home. Miriam asked me to help her do some weeding in the yard. I went to the yard. I picked the weeds. Time passed. Miriam went to the store to get some groceries. A bleak unreal feeling overcame me. I remembered what Holst had said: *I won't feel anything.*

V

Mars

Home, Safe, Warm

Years passed. By the time I reached my late teens, almost nothing remained of the life Mum, Dad, Sebastian, and I had once shared on Cannon Road. Even my memories were scrambled and fragmentary. I could recall glimpses of the time Before, the early childhood world of the garden and the Jungle and the four of us standing on the summit of Slieve Donard, but the chaos that had succeeded it was so disruptive to my memory, I sometimes wondered if there had ever been a time in reality when the separate broken parts of our family formed a whole. Before was like Atlantis, a legendary lost continent, long ago collapsed into the sea. In the absence of tangible evidence, its existence was easy to dismiss as a childish fable. But still there were those who claimed that the storied civilization had existed in objective reality. "No, you didn't imagine it—she was lovely," my father said, recalling my mother prior to her transformation.

The past made no sense. I resolved to put it behind me. I focused on moving forward: running ahead. I devoted the following decade, from my late teens to my late twenties, to creating an impersonation of a functional human being, building enough of an outer shell of book smarts to convince the world—and myself—that I was *someone*, that I knew what I was doing, that I understood how to live. I got into the University of Oxford. After college, I got a job as a researcher and then a producer of British network television documentaries. I spent six weeks in Papua New Guinea for the Discovery Channel, flying by helicopter to remote jungle villages. I sought out the hardest challenges I could find, priding myself on my ability to survive anything, to accomplish anything, proving that there was nothing I couldn't do. Meanwhile the chaos of my childhood and my mother's ongoing illness remained a mystery I felt powerless to solve. I seldom spoke about what happened to my family in the mid-1980s. I never sought therapy. Fear and shame pursued me like a shadow that was impossible for me ever to outrun. I medicated the feelings with alcohol, marijuana, MDMA, and LSD. On MDMA, I experienced an overwhelming sense of bliss in which I no longer felt like an isolated mind, painfully separate from the world beyond the frontiers of my skin, but instead lovingly interconnected with others. Yet when the drug wore off, the pain of isolation felt even greater.

I hadn't understood my parents' psychotic breakdowns when they occurred: the experiences had utterly transcended my teenage understanding. They started to become clear in hindsight, through successive cycles of remembering, but never with any sense of finality or closure. I tried to remember; I couldn't remember. I tried to run away from my mother and never think about her again; my route was a circle that always took me back to her.

During the winter vacation of my second year at Oxford I took LSD with my friend Ned at his parents' cottage in the English countryside. The next day we had breakfast in a café. The locals called it the Nostril. A large main room connected to a smaller room at the back, like a narrowing office, and the walls throughout were painted red, curving in at the edges. I could understand why the café had earned its unofficial name: it was easy to imagine that I was sitting inside a giant nose. I felt calm. In my hallucinatory state, it occurred to me that the organ in which I had found myself was not a nostril after all but somewhere much deeper inside. The womb. A realization dawned on me: *My mother is dead.*

I recognized the thought as the formulation in words of wordless knowledge I had borne in a bodily ache for a very long while, a realization I had until then succeeded in screening from conscious recognition, because of the shattering grief that came from rendering her loss explicit in my mind.

I wasn't delusional. I understood the death was not a physical one. The thought connected to an awareness, for the first time with clarity, of grief. She was gone. After enduring her verbal assaults, and then witnessing psychosis engulf her mind, I had severed myself from the memory of the emotional force field that had once bound the two of us as one. I was alone. I realized that I had been alone for a very long time. But this clarity gave way to confusion in reconciling my impression of her psychological demise with my understanding of her physical continuity. *Who, then, has died?* I wondered.

Sometimes I fantasized that she would suffer a fatal accident or terminal cancer. I would picture a cute girl noticing me in a pub and seeing my sad face and inquiring about my sadness, to which I would respond, *My mum died,* and I would see the sympathy in Cute Girl's eyes. It would be so much easier, I imagined, to bear a grief so much more comprehensible, a loss that other people could understand. All the other words I could think of—*She's mad*—fell short of communicating my bereavement. *I must be evil,* I'd think, catching myself in the fantasy of a car wreck or metastatic brain cancer, as if my mind had murdered her. And along with my ambiguous sense of loss came another problem: how to conceive of the identity of the woman with my mother's legal name who sent me deranged postcards every week. *Who are you, Mrs. Thompson? You seem to know things about me. You seem to mention places that I once visited with my mother. Are you a friend of hers, or perhaps a distant relation? I do wish you would refrain from signing your postcards "Mum"—I find it so very confusing.*

I can remember glancing at the scrawl on one of her postcards, the loops and curls of her dense cursive inscribed so tightly together that the words joined in places, forming the equivalent of massive compound nouns, and it struck me that I and my childhood self were twins, two beings sharing the same body at different times, grown-up Thompson sailing off on the ship of consciousness while little-boy me drifted toward the faraway island of childhood memory. *Why are these words so unbearable to me? Is it the outdated references or the disjointed prose or the eccentric punctuation?* It was all of that: the disconnection, the lack of acknowledgment for our family's collapse, the impression conveyed in the postcards that her own demise was unknown to her. *Don't you know that I know you're not my actual mother?* There were lines between us, my mother and my father and my brother and myself, Clara and Mummy, a little boy and whoever I had now become, umbilical cords connecting past and present, but in my mother's mind they were tangled, broken, stitched together in shabby scraps. *Here are the scraps*, she seemed to be saying in her postcards. *You piece them together.* But I couldn't, or wouldn't. *Why the hell should I? You're the one who tore us apart.*

But I felt troubled by this impression I had of two women, my mother and Mrs. Thompson, that it was surely a sort of convenient fiction I told myself so I wouldn't have to go home for Christmas. Was there something unique about her metamorphosis that diverged in any meaningful way from the transformations that occur to all phenomena that have existed in time? We cannot step in the same river twice, Heraclitus told us. A little boy turns into a man: Were those two selves not likewise mutually distinct, separated in space and time, unlike in mind and body? And even in the present, it occurred to me, *Am I not this very moment a crowd of conflicting thoughts? Is there really a still point in all this flux, a core me?* No, I was a fiction too, so it wasn't at all clear to me that my mother was any different, rendering my loss of her all the more confusing: I was mourning somebody still alive.

"DID YOUR FATHER TELL you where he was going?" she said. He had. Oslo. He'd met a Norwegian woman on a Gaelic language course in Dublin, fallen in love with her, and gone to live with her in Norway. He insisted to me that he'd been explicit that he meant leaving her forever and told her he had met someone else and was going to live with her in Norway. Either he hadn't been explicit or she hadn't understood, or she didn't want to understand. "He's in Oslo. I thought he told you." She said, "No, he didn't. And he's not allowed. It's criminal."

I understood why he wanted to leave. She was impossible. I wanted to leave too. But I couldn't. Or wouldn't. I wasn't sure. *How come Dad gets to leave, but not me?* It was a double bind. Weeks would pass and I'd try to forget all about her. Then she would call me at work and start droning on. I'd listen for a while, but then I couldn't stand it. I felt like she wasn't talking to *me*; that she could just as easily have gone on blathering if some random stranger had picked up the phone. I'd hang up, then feel guilty for not caring more, and worried she might have said something important that I missed while I spaced out as she was droning on. I couldn't bear the thought of her, all alone, crazy and desperate. But I couldn't talk to her either. I went on circling around like this—from guilt to caring to trying to talk to failing to spacing out and not caring and then back to guilt—for years.

For several years after my father left my mother, she struggled to comprehend that his departure was permanent. In my mother's phone calls and letters to me, she characterized him as a sort of international fugitive; she had informed INTERPOL, the British Embassy, and the BBC about his criminal act of desertion, she said. She seemed compelled by forces outside her control on a downward spiral toward destitution. My father had left her with a flat in a pleasant neighborhood in Belfast. About a year following his departure, she sold the flat in Belfast and moved to England, then Ireland, then England again, depleting her capital in each impulsive move. One time I called the Realtor, hoping to block the sale. I sent a fax with a five-paragraph essay that would have made my Oxford tutors proud, arguing my case. The sale defied all reason, I explained. All her running back and forth, every reckless movement, should be construed as a message to my father, I argued. *You did this to me*, one should imagine my mother wishing my father to understand, I told the Realtor. "In conclusion, it thus becomes incumbent upon me, and I respectfully submit to you, sir," I wrote, or formal-sounding words to that effect, "to take action to disrupt my mother's self-destructive downward spiral: please don't let her sell the house." I can remember the Realtor expressing sympathy for my concern but also an understanding of her freedom as an adult person to do as she pleased.

One day in the winter she called to say that her neighbors in an adjacent flat had discovered a carbon monoxide leak. I told her to turn off her heater. "It's too cold," she said. I called the company that maintained the heaters in the area. I warned the person on the phone that unless someone checked my mother's heater, she might die. "Old lady, is she, your mum?" the person said. "Yes," I said. She was middle-aged. But saying she was old was a kind of idiom for what I couldn't say out loud, couldn't even think, didn't have the words for. I understood that mental illness was involved. Back then I wasted a lot of time wondering what particular psychiatric jargon best matched her idiosyncrasies. *Is it schizophrenia? But isn't that when people hear voices? I don't THINK that sounds like her. . . . But could it be? What if she hears voices and never tells anyone about them? Keeps her delusions to herself? But she was never shy of speaking. . . . Surely if she thought aliens were beaming signals into her brain she'd have told me all about it? So if not schizophrenia, what is it? What the hell is wrong with her? What happened to her? To US?*

My mother was in her mid-fifties. Yet I can remember my impression that I had no choice but to call her old. Her fragility did not derive from her chronological age, but I lacked the words to say what was actually wrong with her. I shared my mother's sense of abandonment and anger at Dad. *Call yourself a father? You were supposed to protect us. You failed back when I really needed you, and now you're doing it again.* We spoke about once a month on the phone. I can remember my feelings of contempt— how after an incident like my intervention with the heating company, it seemed to me that I was taking on responsibilities that neither of us wanted but which in my opinion surely belonged to him, not me. "I don't understand why I have to do all of this for her," I told him one time. "But you don't," he said. "Someone else could." "What do you mean, *someone?*" I said. "There are people who do that sort of thing," he said.

I knew he meant social services. He wasn't wrong. There likely could have been ways that someone other than me might have engaged those services to support someone with needs approximating my mother's. But at the time, I wasn't interested in finding *people who do that sort of thing*—I was furious about the person who from my wounded and resentful perspective had never done the right thing. *That would be you, Dad.*

I wasn't sure which feeling was the worst, contempt or sadness or shame or fear or guilt, or all of the bad feelings mixed together. I railed at the injustice of my plight. *Why me? I'm in my twenties. I'm not supposed to have to deal with things like this. Sure, maybe when you're middle-aged your parents end up in nursing homes or whatever and you have to look after them. But not now, when I'm so young. And where the hell did Dad go? How come he gets to skip off to his new life in Norway and I'm stuck here cleaning up his mess?*

I felt angry with my father for a long time. I resented him for failing to protect Sebastian and me, for failing to get help. *Why don't* you *do something?* His words from those mad days in Fairgreen Road formed a loop in my memory. *How absurd*, I would think, that he could have imagined that, of the two of us, not he but I—a fifteen-year-old boy at the time—should have been the one to find some way of helping Mum, as if our responsibilities in the family as father and son were equivalent, or even reversed. *You did this to us*, I would think. But over time my anger faded. I forgave him. I felt compassion for the suffering he had endured. I came to understand that he had done his best with the emotional resources available to him. He had tried to get Mum to see our family doctor; he had tried to persuade her to participate in family therapy. Her answer always had been no. She—or her illness—was an implacable force. In the end, he had given up trying. I came to understand what a crushing loss that was for him, how my anger at him after our family collapsed was a measure of how much I had loved the miraculous Daddy I remembered from my early childhood. I hadn't lost Mummy—we all had. Including my mother herself.

I felt no anger toward her. Her disturbance was so extreme, it had the quality of a natural disaster. Does anyone resent a hurricane? Instead I felt survivor's guilt, the painful knowledge that while I had survived our family's implosion and moved on with my life, with each passing year she seemed to be descending further into isolation and destitution in a downward spiral I was powerless to stop. And I felt sadness, shame, loneliness, and grief.

I didn't want to feel those emotions. At the time, for the most part, I couldn't even have discerned my inchoate bad feelings with discrete names. I knew I didn't want to feel whatever it was I was feeling. I understood there were two ways of blocking out the bad feelings: Ecstasy and terror. When I took a pill in a dance club, I could feel my separate self dissolve into the lights and music. I could imagine all the people, living life in peace. When I rode my racing bike in twelfth gear through dense commuter traffic in the dark or when I shimmied hundreds of feet up vertical rock walls, the universe outside the frontier of the next five seconds fell away, leaving only the present second's wide-eyed panting imperative not to fall. But then I would return to my flat and sit at my desk and remember the Jungle and the garden and feel sad.

Once in a while I'd get a phone call or letter from Sebastian. He was in London for a while, somewhere on the outer reaches of the Northern Line, too far for me to bother ever going to visit, then Lyon, Brussels, Vienna. Meanwhile, Mum moved from Dublin to Belfast, then Southampton, Belfast again, Southampton again, Istanbul, then Southampton.

When now and then I would catch up with Sebastian in his latest foreign country, the conversation would soon drift to crazy stories from Cannon Road. There was a solace of sorts in reassembling the broken pieces of our respective memories into more coherent whole stories; in recalling how lost we both had felt, how strange and awful it had been for us to experience the explosion of our family into four isolated parts, separated now by hundreds of miles across the earth, each one of us struggling for the most part alone to remember how that explosion had occurred.

..

The forest is as black as bat wings. My mood has shifted. I'm scared. I don't like the dark now. *I wonder if she is waiting for me. I wonder if she will leave me.* I have to remind myself where I am: a forest trail on a mountain, a path that has an ending. At the top of this climb is Brockway Summit, the mile-50 aid station, where I'll take a short nap. Miriam will be there, I know. I trust her. There is absolutely no way she'd ever let me down. Let's say for some unforeseeable reason she can't make it. The car breaks down, say. Even then, I'll be totally fine. There are people at Brockway. Friendly, generous people who can help me. I have a drop bag there. I can eat and drink and lie down on one of the cots for a while and everything will be fine. So if I think about it, there's really nothing to worry about. The scared feeling must be coming from somewhere outside any conscious thought. Somewhere deeper. Older. Primordial. Sometime when the darkness was an absence, not a presence. When the world outside was frightening and silent.

ABOUT A HUNDRED FEET up ahead I can see fairy lights in a clearing. I see cars and people and tents hung with fairy lights. Brockway. Mile 50. I hear Miriam call my name. I see her smiling face.

I sit down. She brings me a plate of food. I eat the food. I take off my shoes. I've been on my feet for around fifteen hours and awake for the past eighteen. I need a nap. Miriam has laid down sleeping bags for both of us. We lie on the ground next to each other. "Home, safe, warm," she says. "Yes," I say.

Home, safe, warm. Miriam was first to say this. It was a few years ago. We were hiking in the wilderness. It was dark and cold. We were tired and needed to rest. We were far from camp. "Home . . . safe . . . warm," she said. I repeated her words like a mantra: *home . . . safe . . . warm.*

Mantras are sacred sounds designed to help those who say them remember their deepest purpose or values. *Home, safe, warm* helps Miriam and me remember that we have committed ourselves as a refuge to each other. Say one of us is freaking out. There's a bill to pay but no money in the bank. There's a report due tomorrow, but now it's midnight and we have to sleep. Forests on fire. The world on fire. Then one of us says the magic words. *Home, safe, warm. We'll get through this. I'm here for you.* Almost any trail or trial in life is traversable when you have that feeling of sanctuary. Someplace that feels like home. The place doesn't have to be physical. It's a state of mind. *Someone* who feels like home. The person who really knows you and loves you and you can lie on the ground with and hold and you know that everything is going to be fine.

I lie down and close my eyes. I can hear loud rock music playing in the tent. Memories of moving through the forest all day form a green tunnel in my semiconscious mind through which I experience a feeling of disembodied running. The green tunnel leads into music that sounds farther away now and into which my consciousness seems to enter. I feel the warmth and love of Miriam beside me and know that I am home and safe and warm. I see foxes and smiling bears in the imaginary forest. I know the dream forest as a dream. I can feel the friendship of the trees and hear their happy laughter. *Home safe warm . . . home safe warm . . .*

The Hands of Thetis

There is a rhythm in all things: an intrinsic tendency for ordered systems to reproduce a familiar equilibrium. Consider the thermostat. It has two key components: a thermometer and a switch. Set the thermostat for 70 and when the temperature dips to 65 the heat comes on until the air hits 70 again. And thus a comfortable temperature stays constant. Consider the amoeba. It interacts with the environment to re-create its nucleus and cell wall. Now scale this principle of self-perpetuation from a single-celled organism to the hundred billion neurons of the human brain. The intricate architecture of our neural thermostats underlies every aspect of our existence as conscious creatures on Earth whose survival depends on a certain amount of predictability. We depend on a degree of order, for instance, in the availability of food, water, shelter, and social contact. But chaos can become its own kind of order. We run back to disaster to remind ourselves that we're strong enough to bear it. Human tragedy is circular, a rhythm that can pull us back into the same old chaos, over and over again. Unconscious forces draw us back to the edge of the precipice. We have been here before, it seems, standing above the abyss, with no memory of ever choosing to come here, as if the abyss made the decision for us. This is why Oedipus kills his dad and weds his mom: he doesn't know who he really is. We are blind to our true nature. "The patient does not remember anything of what he has forgotten and repressed, but acts it out," wrote Freud.[11] "He reproduces it not as a memory but an action; he repeats it, without, of course, knowing that he is repeating it." When Achilles was an infant, his mother, Thetis, a half-divine being, bathed him in the magical waters of the Underground. She held him by his foot. The magic water rendered Achilles almost invincible: he became so fast on his feet, it was said, he could outrun a deer. Yet held in his mother's hands, part of Achilles was vulnerable. Neither son nor mother knew this. Thetis was half-human, after all, not an all-seeing goddess. We are all Achilles. We are all in the hands of Thetis, compelled by forces outside of our awareness, never fully separate from the relationships that hold us, the human beings and historical forces and physical processes that brought us into being, from the double helix molecules that compose the human genome to the structure of our families and civilization.

IN THE THIRTY MINUTES that Miriam left me doing chores in the front yard, a day after my return from the hospital, my mind unraveled. On the psych ward, I had erroneously concluded that inpatient hospitalization was doing nothing for me. But on the ward, I was always surrounded by other people. And I couldn't have acted on suicidal thoughts even if I'd wanted to.

I was aware of my pain and its ostensible sole remedy. The question in my mind concerned the moment of its ending. I understood the consequential character of the action I was now contemplating. I knew that I stood at the threshold of annihilation. I would be gone forever. I didn't contemplate what it might be like for Miriam to discover my dead body. I didn't wonder how Sebastian or Mum or Dad or anyone who had known and cared about me would ever absorb the knowledge that I had killed myself. I couldn't imagine the unseen threads that bound my soul to others near and far or the rupture felt in the human fabric when one of us cuts their thread and vanishes, the agony for those left behind, all the questions that would never be answered, grieving a life incomplete and now forever beyond completion.

No such thoughts occurred to me. All I could think about was my horrible pain and my wish for it to end. The past was gone. The future was gone. Hope, faith, the idea of anything ever changing: gone, gone, gone. Then something else was gone. Me. I felt like I wasn't really *me* anymore. Everything felt unreal, like a scene in a movie.

You know that part in a movie when it's near the end? You don't need to check the actual number of minutes on the screen. You can tell you're in the final act from where you are in the story. The war is almost over. The explosions can't get any louder. It's obvious now what's going to happen. The ending might be ten seconds away or maybe it gets dragged out through a series of false crescendos. But either way, the end is almost here.

That's how I felt. I was watching the saddest movie in the world. The one in which the hero dies at the end and the hero was me.

One day when I was about fifteen I found myself in the passenger seat of our family car while my mother screamed at me. Years later all I could remember was the venomous tone of her voice and the feeling inside that I was hated. *Please make it stop*, I thought, but her screaming would not stop. She screamed and screamed and screamed, and I felt hated and hated and hated, until I turned into a hateful thing.

I opened the car door. The road sped beneath me in a gray blur. I felt a hand on my shoulder, and I heard my mother calling my name and shouting, "No!" Her rage had disappeared. In its place was a voice that sounded caring and concerned. I had stopped being a hateful thing. I had turned back into a boy.

By threatening to destroy myself, I had reminded her of the part of her that loved me. Her screaming stopped, and the loving mother I could recall from my earlier childhood appeared in place of the troubled, raging person she had become. We drove home in silence and never spoke of the incident again. Looking back, the memory had the sovereign quality of a separate island of the mind, severed altogether from anything that came before or after it, a runaway instant of experience outside of linear time.

Once moments of experience become runaways like that, they tend to keep on running. It's hard to make sense of them, learn from them, or bind them together in a linear recollection of the passage of time, so they fade into history. In the outer world of physical reality, I opened the car door sometime in the mid-1980s, in my teens. But in the inner world of the psyche, no time had passed between the moment I opened the car door in England and the moment I left the front yard in San Francisco, with the noise of screaming still echoing through my mind, and walked into the kitchen.

I took all the liquor bottles out of the pantry. I picked up a camping knife. I lined up the bottles on the kitchen table. I drank half a bottle of tequila and a quart of aquavit. The hateful feeling faded with every swig of liquor. I staggered to the bathroom. I opened the cabinet. I took out a bottle of Klonopin. I poured the pills onto the palm of my hand. *Twenty pills: it ought to be enough.* I put the plug in the bathtub. I turned the faucet on. While the water was running, I went back to the kitchen. I drank a few big gulps of aquavit. I went back to the bathroom. *This is what it feels like for someone to die by suicide*, I thought. I took off my clothes. I could see that my legs were trembling. I got into the tub. I remembered the actions that I now intended to perform. *See the wall: soon there will be no such thing as walls or seeing. Feel the water: soon there will be no such thing as water or feeling. Move the fingers of the hand: soon there will be no such thing as hands and nothing moving.* I swallowed the pills. I reached for the knife.

VI

Jupiter

Remembering Everything
and Nothing

Lights. Is this death? No. I am thinking. Conscious. Alive. I woke in one of those blue backless gowns they give you in the ER. I was lying on a hospital bed, in the little sphere of privacy formed by the blue curtains on either side of me. *How odd to feel so chipper*, I thought, floating in the Christmas morning euphoria induced by a fistful of Klonopin, a mood I could see didn't match the somber faces around me. Miriam. Miriam's brother Matt. A couple of nurses. Miriam was sitting at the foot of the bed, leafing through *The Noonday Demon* by Andrew Solomon. Her brother was in the chair beside her. "Hi, guys," I said. "Go back to sleep," said Miriam. "How are you doing, Matt?" I asked her brother. "I just feel bad for Miriam," he said.

Miriam had come home several hours earlier that afternoon to find me sitting on the couch, reading *People* magazine. "I said hello, and you started talking, and this gibberish came out of your mouth," she told me, much later. "You were slurring your words. I knew you'd been drinking, but I had no idea how much. There was no sign of the liquor bottles—you must have put them away. I said, 'Honey, are you drunk?' and you told me you'd gone to the bar and had a couple of beers with Ned, and I thought, *Oh, good. He's seeing his friends again. He must be getting better*, and for a minute I actually thought it was all kind of funny, the way you were talking gibberish in that slurry way. But then you tried to get up to go to the bathroom, but you were stumbling about, and when you got to the bathroom you puked your guts out. It was obvious you were totally smashed. Not two-beers-with-your-buddy drunk. Falling-down-crazy-paralytic drunk. I got scared. I called your social worker. She said, 'Get him in the shower and put him into bed and don't freak out too much. He's starting our outpatient program in the morning.' I told you to get in the shower. You were so drunk you couldn't take off your own pants. There was no way I was going to be able to get you undressed and lift you into the tub all by myself. You're too heavy. I called Matt to come over and help me. Matt came over real fast, and I turned on the shower and we got you undressed, and the moment we had your pants off I saw your leg and then I just lost it. It was all bloody and there were cuts all over it with this one really big slash down your right thigh. It was fucking horrific. I panicked and called 911, and they took you to the ER."

THE OLDEST SURVIVING REFERENCES to the legend of Atlantis occur in two of Plato's late dialogues, *Timaeus* and *Critias*. A long time ago, wrote Plato, Atlantis was a peaceful state. But the Atlanteans fell victim to the dark side of their nature. Plato concludes *Critias* with an account of how Zeus then decided to intervene to save the Atlanteans from their own worst instincts.

Zeus was the king of Olympus, the son of Cronus, the god of time, the grandson of Gaia and Uranus, the primordial deities of earth and air. In Rome they called him Jupiter. Zeus knew everything that could be known. *Critias* ends as follows:

> *Zeus, the god of gods, who rules according to law, and is able to see into such things, perceiving that an honorable race was in a woeful plight, and wanting to inflict punishment on them, that they might be chastened and improve, collected all the gods into their most holy habitation, which, being placed in the center of the world, beholds all created things. And when he had called them together, he spake as follows:—*[12]

The text runs out into the void. The rest of *Critias* is presumed lost. What Zeus said in his effort to save Atlantis is unknown. But maybe Plato had nothing to say. Maybe Zeus had nothing to say.

I WOKE WITH NO recollection whatsoever of anything that happened in the four hours that elapsed between the moment I swallowed the pills with the expectation that I would soon be dead and the moment I woke in the hospital still alive. That time is a void in my memory. In the strange twilight of suicidal consciousness in which my actions seemed to unfold with the unreal, unwilled quality of a dream, I entered an alien zone of experience where I was no longer *I*. Insofar as this not-I shared anything with the original I it once had been, my former selfhood, now shrunken into silence, it was the anguished recognition of loss, a kind of grief for the feeling of being someone, now gone, forever gone. I wanted out. I wanted to run away from being a dark mass of pain, trapped in the hellish circle of thoughts going round and round and leading nowhere, the fear and shame and sadness that had spiraled downward and abandoned me outside time, the nobody that I had become.

But something had stopped me from following through on my plan. *I won't feel anything*—I had remembered Holst's words. I was going to get blind drunk, then open up a vein in my arm. But I had initiated this plan with the knowledge that Miriam would soon be coming back. The plan left open at least a possibility that I might be found and helped before death became inevitable. Maybe I tried to cut my arm and missed. Maybe I then saw the horrible reality of bleeding flesh. My flesh. My body. Me. Maybe in seeing and feeling the wound on my leg, no one turned into someone, not-I back into I. *This isn't a dream*, perhaps I thought. *This is reality. I could die.* Maybe, restored by fear to some vestige of self-awareness, I realized who and where I was, and could picture the ghastly scene unfolding through Miriam's imagined eyes, so I put on a show like everything was normal. By the time she came home, I had drained the tub and put all the liquor bottles back into the cabinet.

So many maybes. It's impossible to say for certain what chaotic thoughts occurred to me during that void in memory. But one thing is clear: part of me still wanted to live. I had thought that I wanted to die. But I was much more than my thoughts. I was my feet and thighs, my breath and beating heart, the wordless knowledge still within me of the power to get up, move forward, and survive. *I* wanted to die. But my body wanted to live. My legs had always led me from disaster.

THE NEXT MORNING I woke to find myself in bed in the ward in my blue hospital pajamas and top, back in the same room with the Prisoner and Rip Van Winkle as if I had never left. I still felt high from the Klonopin.

I'm not supposed to feel so chipper. I tried to kill myself!

After breakfast I went and stood by the pay phone and paced back and forth, unsure what etiquette demanded in my circumstances. "I'm sorry," I said. "How could you do that to someone you love?" Miriam said, and hung up. *But I'm not sure it was really me.* Not that I had anyone else to blame.

I called Sebastian. "Why don't you think about someone other than yourself?" he said. "What would have happened if you'd succeeded? You'd have damaged me and Dad and Mum irreparably."

"I know," I said.

"But what if it happens again?"

"It won't," I said.

"But you said that before. When I called you. Miriam told me you were suicidal, and I asked you if you'd ever actually do it, and you said no, it was just a feeling."

"That was true, then," I said, "but I won't do it again. I'm feeling a bit better now."

"But how am I supposed to believe you? How do you know you won't feel worse again?"

I didn't know what to tell him. *He's right. I might feel worse again.* Sebastian asked me if I needed anything in the hospital. "Sheet music," I said.

About an hour later a nurse handed me some faxed pages of piano music. "From your brother," she said. It was a piece by Oscar Peterson called "Hymn to Freedom." I sat in the dayroom for hours, playing the first five bars over and over again.

DR. BROWNING DIDN'T EXACTLY look thrilled to see me. I could get why she was mad. Imagine some Goody-Two-Shoes whose lifetime worst screw-up was a single B minus in sixth grade, staking her name and reputation and legal liability on the disheveled Englishman who swore up and down he no longer posed a grave danger to himself only to find him back on the ward in less than forty-eight hours with self-inflicted knife wounds: Who could blame her if she hated me a bit? I had told her that I didn't intend to act upon my recurrent thoughts of suicide. This wasn't false. It wasn't true either. Perhaps that sounds crazy. But this is how that logic goes: The two problems in the statement are *I* and *intend*. Say you intend to do something. Normally an intention tends to last a bit longer than, say, the five seconds it takes for the words to come out of your mouth. *I intend to order the chocolate mousse for dessert*: no one cares if you change your mind. *I intend to feed your dog*: it matters to the dog and dog owner if you follow through. But when the doctor asked me about my suicidal intentions, it felt more like the chocolate mousse sort of intention. Any second I might feel differently and change my mind. The *I* that said I wasn't going to act on suicidal thoughts and the *I* that acted on them were not the same *I*. I'd told Miriam that being stuck inside the hospital wasn't helping me in any way whatsoever. But I was wrong. Hospitalization had indeed helped me. It had stopped me from trying to kill myself.

The doctor handed me a piece of paper she had printed out from a medical website. It described an illness called borderline personality disorder. Its symptoms were "emotional instability," "feelings of worthlessness," "impulsive behavior," and "impaired relationships." *Doesn't everyone feel like that?* I wondered. The description referred to the borderline patient's "frantic efforts to thwart real or imagined abandonment" and the tendency of individuals thus afflicted to self-induce physical injuries to stimulate chemical responses in the body that can reduce emotional pain.

"Does this sound like you, Mr. Thompson?" she said. "I thought it might fit, because of the cutting."

The cutting: I had indeed cut myself. I had cut myself off from the land where I was born. I had acquired a way of coping with life by severing my mind from difficult experiences. It wasn't far-fetched for Dr. Browning to see the gash on my leg and hear about the chaos of my adolescence and match these two pieces of information with the criteria for a disorder that included similar features. Still, I experienced our interaction about *the cutting* as strange and distancing. There is nothing wrong with reductionism. To explain or understand almost any phenomenon necessarily means attending to the important parts of it, and neglecting others. To do otherwise would be like asking someone for directions to a street address and hearing them describe every square inch of the road and the molecular composition of asphalt. The person who gave street directions in such a manner would be giving an answer at the wrong level of explanation. Dr. Browning's interpretation of my knife wound and family history as perhaps symptomatic of borderline personality traits was a coherent formulation, on its surface. But it is worth asking what this explanation accomplished. Did it yield more information than was already self-evident? No. I had cut my own leg; I felt worthless. And diagnosis was its own kind of violence. It cut me down to a set of disease criteria. It cut out how I felt on the inside. It cut out meaning. In different ways both of us were cutters, Dr. Browning and I.

AROUND TEN AT NIGHT the nurses turned the television off. It was quiet on the ward. Most nights I would see one or two lonely souls wandering about the empty corridors. I sat down, leaning against a wall, and took out a scrap of paper. I drew a line down the page like one of the coun-selors had told me to, dividing it into two columns, one for pro and the other for con. I tried to think of how to divide the loop running through my head into two and tell the difference between pros and cons when the whole problem was not being able to say that one thing was really any bet-ter than another, because the moment something felt like a pro, all I could think of was how it was really a con, and vice versa, so everything went round and round from pro to con and back to pro until it turned into pro-con-pro-con-pro-con. One evening, as I sat on the floor, lost in thought, a young woman with long dark hair, wearing a robe over her blue hospital pajamas, wandered past and then sat down next to me.

"What are you writing?" she said.

"Nothing," I said. I showed her the page with the line on it and the words *pro* and *con* at the top. "I can't write anything anymore."

"Why are you here?" she said.

"I tried to kill myself," I said.

"How?" she said.

"With booze and pills and a knife," I said.

"Can I see?" she said.

I hitched up my hospital pajamas. She saw the long red gash that ex-tended from my right hip to my kneecap.

Her face scrunched up with a look of revulsion. "Oh Jesus, that's fuckin' horrible," she said. "How could you do that to yourself? Oh, dude—I mean what the fuck, that's just fuckin' gross."

She looked about nineteen. She still lived at home with her mom and dad, she said. They called 911 when she took a bunch of pills. "I'm al-ways doing shit like that," she said. She got mad and told her parents she wished she'd never been born. The whole world was fuckin' stupid, so why bother? The only thing that helped was painting. She made screen-print T-shirts and had a little business selling them to other kids. The name of her business was Invisible Laserbeam.

"Why can't you write anything?" she said.

"My head goes round and round," I said. "Nothing makes sense when it comes out. Just random words."

"What's wrong with random words?" she said. "A poem is basically random words. Sometimes I write poems. You should try it."

"I like poems," I said.

"Ever write any?" she said.

"I have spread my dreams under your feet . . . Tread softly because you tread on my dreams . . ."

"Write that shit down, dude."

"It's Yeats," I said. "'Aedh Wishes for the Cloths of Heaven.'"

"Give me that paper."

I gave it to her. In a couple of minutes, she filled the page with a poem entitled "Missing Equivalency":

> Speaking of speaking in times historical
> Documentation has preconceived
> The notion of space to fulfill
> Endlessness in all of the space
> Left to fulfill. Dot, dot, dot. Right?
> Okay, so here's the issue: time being
> Equivalent to space in the respect
> Of absence and some sort of ending.
> "Like I've never wanted out."
> What it's like never knowing,
> What it's like never needing feeling in and out and around the
> Glove that I wear to find sorrow.
> Captivation confusion, letting go,
> Remembrance.
> How can I remember everything
> And nothing at all at the same time?

How can I remember everything and nothing? You got that right, sister. If the doctors had names in their textbooks for the way people like me and Invisible Laserbeam were really feeling, not the wounds on the outside, the signs they sorted into labels, they would listen to her poem. Whatever happened way back in the time before, who knew. People like me and Invisible Laserbeam were never speaking of the time itself but *speaking of speaking in times historical*. We had chronic What It's Like Never Knowing. We had severe Captivation Confusion. We had child-onset What It's Like Never Needing Feeling. You could say such talk had nothing to do with science. You might suppose the brain doctors were working with their chosen organ much like heart doctors evaluate the ticker. There was something broken in folks like me and Invisible, no doubt about it. One day in the future, maybe, someone would make a map of every brain cell, all one hundred billion of them, and every electric signal between them, like a trail map of the forest of the mind. They could follow every thought and feeling and sensation flowing down every single path, like a GPS satellite tracking the motions of runners in the woods from far above, and know when someone was lost, when feelings disappeared in the dark undergrowth in the nighttime, when thoughts ran in circles and never found their way toward meaning anything. But until that day came, there was no map. The doctors looked at what we said and did. There was no blood test for crazy, no brain scan for a wound in the soul. *Frantic efforts to thwart real or imagined abandonment*. Yes. *What it's like never needing feeling*. Yes. *Captivation confusion*, and *never knowing*, and *remembering everything and nothing*: Yes, yes, yes.

I CONTINUED TO EXPERIENCE some relief from my own anguish in my informal role as listener to the suffering of others. I must have looked better on the outside than I felt on the inside. Perhaps it was the English accent, or a quiet demeanor that passed for introversion instead of the maelstrom of panic and shame and suicidal thinking I was actually ex- periencing. This paradox was sometimes disorienting for others. One evening a young Black woman came in on a gurney, her body shaking in violent convulsions. I saw her the following morning in the dining room. I sat down opposite her. I said hello.

"I'm Naomi," she said. She was eighteen years old, she said. She looked younger. She had frightened eyes and a tremulous voice. She had swallowed about a hundred lithium tablets and half a bottle of vodka the night before, she said. She told her mom. Her mom called 911. She was taken to the ER. The doctors pumped her stomach and then they sent her to the psych ward. Her heart was going *baboom, baboom,* around 180 beats a minute, she said. They couldn't give her any medicine for it because her liver and kidneys couldn't handle it. "The doctors told me I'm lucky to be alive," she said. She took my hand and pressed it to her racing heart. "I'm so lonesome, I could die," she said. I saw her notice the wedding band on my left hand. "Your wife is a lucky lady," she said.

"I don't think so," I said. "One day you'll meet someone too, I bet."

"You think so?"

"Yes," I said.

"You're a wonderful person," she said. "I'll miss you when you're gone. You're going home today, right?"

"No, I just got here," I said.

"Oh," she said, in a disappointed tone, as if I had broken a promise. "You think you know someone. But then you don't."

Naomi didn't know me. Neither did I really know myself. But the staff on the ward continued to do their best to make sense of my self-destructive behavior. The folks who ran the meeting at seven in the library always brought chocolate cookies, one of the nurses told me. "Real big chocolate cookies. And you should definitely go. I don't think I need to tell you why." I was about to say that he did need to tell me when I remembered that I had wound up in the hospital after washing down a fistful of Klonopin with an entire bottle of hard liquor. *Okay, I get where you're coming from,* I thought. *A patient comes in half-dead after he drinks a whole bottle of tequila, no wonder you think he's some sort of wino.* And sure, I'd drunk a lot over the years. But didn't everyone? I knew that I had problems. But alcoholism surely wasn't one of them.

Alcoholic—the word summoned images of a homeless geezer collapsed on the sidewalk, puking. *I'm not THAT guy. But real big chocolate cookies? Sure, sign me up.*

The meeting was convened by two men from the Hospitals and Institutions committee of Alcoholics Anonymous. One of the men read the preamble and asked me to read the steps. I was the sole patient in attendance. "I don't think I'm an alcoholic," I told the visitor. "The nurse told me I was supposed to come here." I told the visitors about my use of drugs and alcohol. The tall man said, "I don't know either—you might be or you might not be." He gave me a copy of a thick paperback book with a blue cover. "Check it out," he said. "You might find some of it interesting. Especially the stories." After the meeting, I went and sat in the corridor and opened the book.

He was right about the stories. Reading the book, I understood that my image of an alcoholic as a homeless wino lying in his own piss and vomit on the sidewalk was a misleading stereotype. Alcoholism was an equal opportunity illness. There were alcoholics in every corner of society—from the park bench to Park Avenue, as they say. According to the Big Book, *alcoholism wasn't even about alcohol.* Booze was the symptom. The disease was in the soul.

One of the stories in the Big Book was entitled "The Man Who Mastered Fear." It was written by a man in the Midwest who drank his way through years of crippling anxiety in the era of the Great Depression until he met Dr. Bob, one of AA's founders, and embraced the program, which he credited with saving his life. The words introducing his story were as follows: "He spent eighteen years running away, and then found he didn't have to run."

IN MORNING GROUP THERAPY, the counselors would encourage us to speak about our thoughts. The approach struck me as consistent with what I understood to be a core principle of American positive thinking, the notion that urges the Debby Downers to turn their frowns upside down, derived from the conception of psychological suffering as an outcome of negative thoughts, whose removal or restructuring would form the pathway to mental health, rather along the lines of the directive in a popular 1940s song: *"Accentuate the positive. Eliminate the negative. Latch on to the affirmative. But don't mess with mister in between."* It was consistent too with the entire history of Western philosophy, which likewise proceeds from an emphasis on the efficacy of reason, exemplified by the dialogues between Plato and his teacher, Socrates, in which fundamental life questions about the nature of reality, society, ethics, love, and so on are explored by probing the conventional thoughts held about them. "I think, therefore I am," wrote Descartes. But I didn't think, at least not in a way that felt like coherent thought. Therefore I was not. I was Mr. In Between.

The doctors and nurses did their damnedest to get head cases like me back inside our bodies. Most days they had us draw or paint a picture or play the bongos. They taught us the idea from a school of psychotherapy called DBT that when contemplating a path that appeared to fork in two directions, it was possible to walk down the middle of them. They provided a fridge full of apples. I munched the apples at every opportunity, discovering that one side effect of my antipsychotic medication was a hunger that I could never satiate. I had always had a sweet tooth. I asked Miriam and my two other visitors to bring chocolate.

The first of those two other visitors was Ned. One evening he came to visit bearing a chocolate croissant. He understood in general terms why I was back in the hospital. But Miriam had spared him some of the goriest details. It wasn't altogether clear to him that I had really intended to die. "I did," I told him. "I'm really glad you failed," he said. "Because if you'd succeeded"—his voice cracked with tears—"I'd have been so sad."

Sad. I had heard anger from Miriam and Sebastian. I had heard confusion from Dr. Browning. Ned was the first person from whom I heard sadness. The first person who didn't make me feel like feeling suicidal was a sin that demanded an apology or a weird sickness with a scary label. Ned would miss me if I was gone.

My second visitor was Tara, Ned's wife. They had met about six months after I met Miriam, and he had moved to San Francisco to live with her. She was a performance artist with elfin features and the creative spirit of the sort of person whom I wondered might be an actual elf. When she was in her teens she was involved in a near-fatal car accident. In the midst of the collision she had a strange experience. Time and space dissolved. Everything was one. In the aftermath of the accident, she had no fear of death. No fear of anything at all. Nothing was solid. The only reality was Now. The point of being alive and conscious was to create something magical. She lived immersed in the present so acutely it seemed at times to border on disabling. If she threw a party, she wouldn't do a single thing to clean up her apartment until the guests were arriving. It was nice to see Tara's kind face and hear her wise and gentle voice. I told her about all my worrying and thinking and every single uncertain thing of the million un-certain things in my life and how I didn't know what was going to happen. "That's right!" she said. "You don't know! Anything could happen!"

IT WAS A SUNNY DAY when I followed the other patients and the coun-selors guarding us to the hospital rooftop. Through the high fence that bordered the blacktop to stop us from jumping off the building, I gazed at the city far below and the ocean stretching to the western horizon and far off in the distance the dark green pyramid of Mount Tamalpais. It was the first time I'd been outside in a long while. It felt good to see the horizon. I joined a group of patients throwing a ball, a young Japanese American man who talked to himself all the time—it was constant, this verbatim transcript of every single random private thought—and a tall, white, skinny meth addict who would sob like a little boy in group and make me wish I could still cry and a tall woman who down on the ward walked around with earplugs to block out all the voices she was hearing and who told me she was in telepathic communication with Eminem and had written half his songs.

"Five minutes, guys," said one of the counselors. "Chaos, violence, war, hell," said the Japanese American man. Soon I would be taken back down below. I knew I wouldn't see the sky again for many hours or even days. Not until the next exercise break tomorrow. Assuming tomorrow was a weekday. Monday through Friday they took us upstairs for thirty minutes on the blacktop in the afternoon. But Saturday and Sunday, they kept us down below. The counselors went home to their families, and the only staff who stuck around were the nurses. You were lucky if you saw a doctor for more than a couple of minutes to ask how you were feeling on your latest psych med cocktail and how much would you still really rather be dead and gone than go on living. What day it was, who knew.

Run, I thought. *Run before it's too late and you're stuck down there. Right now. Run.*

I set off at a sprint from the basketball hoop to the other end of the blacktop, and then back and forth, over and over again, until I could feel my chest moving up and down with each explosion of my breath; feel the beads of sweat forming on my forehead and then dripping down my face; feel the sensation of fast motion through space, see how my thoughts fell silent as my feet pounded on the ground, how the exertion became a kind of tangible bodily pain that soothed the intangible wound in my soul, a good hurt that filled in the aching abyss where the feeling of being *me* once had been; feel how the ground one step ahead of me transformed into ground underfoot, solid and undeniable, reminding me of all the parts that lived and moved in me that had nothing to do with thought. I kept on running until the counselors led me back to the ward.

The Ground Does the Thinking

My eyes open a few seconds before my alarm goes off. As a night's sleep goes, two hours is about as minimal as you can get. But even this short kip has worked wonders on my brain. I feel totally rested and awake. I'm in a good mood and excited to get back on the trail. All of the head fuzziness and weird uncanny fears I was feeling just a couple of hours ago before I lay down are completely gone. It is really astonishing what sleep can do. No wonder insomnia drives people absolutely nuts and torturers use sleep deprivation as a weapon.

I don't have any clear recall of what I dreamed in the brief stretch of kip I've just woken up from. But I know I did dream. None of the images have stayed with me on waking. But I have a vague recollection of my mind becoming this crazy psychedelic maelstrom, like a Disneyland ride on LSD, and of my lucidity now upon waking as the outcome of the dreamworld chaos that preceded it, like calm waters after a storm's swept through. I get out of my sleeping bag and sit on a camping chair while Miriam goes to get me a plate of food from the aid station. I clean my feet. I change my socks. Miriam returns from the tent. "Thank you," I say. "Bye, darling," she says. We kiss goodbye. I run down the trail that leads me back into the forest. In the cool air, with a clear head and a belly full of food and the feeling of Miriam's love still wrapped around me, I fly along the trail as it leads downhill through the beckoning darkness of the forest. It's about four in the morning.

The sun rises. I pass several runners. I wish everyone good morning. I mean it. The morning really is good. It might well be the best morning I've ever had. I reach the top of a steep hill from which the route descends several hundred feet to a road on the kind of narrow, rough-hewn path, strewn with rocks and tree roots, zigzagging through waist-high bushes and little trees, that a reasonable person would navigate with caution. But right now I'm far from reasonable: run far enough on minimal sleep, and reason gives way to a dreamy flow of feeling. I leap down the mountain, flinging my body left and right like a downhill ski racer.

Everything is moving. I have the sense of the ground rushing beneath me at a speed that exceeds my capacity to make any conscious decision. I have disappeared. The captain of the conscious ship of selfhood, the I, the planner and rememberer, surrenders his command post. Mind and body are being propelled by deeper forces. One might say that I stop running, because there is no I. What emerges is two feet dancing, root to rock, a sudden turn, the impression of Earth itself as running. I don't need to think about how I'll get down the mountain. Sometimes you don't need to think about the ground. The ground does the thinking for you.

THE STEEP DESCENT ENDS at a cul-de-sac about three hundred vertical feet above Lake Tahoe. I'm back in civilization. The asphalt feels artificial and alien. I sit down on a curb to take care of my feet. I take off my shoes and shake out all the dust and pebbles and little sticks and bits of foliage. I take my time cleaning my blackened feet with alcohol wipes. I dress one or two small blisters between my toes. I dry my feet with baby powder. I put on a fresh pair of socks. The course markers lead me down the road to the edge of the lake. As I walk along the road, I can see a caravan of haggard ultrarunners marching on the sidewalk ahead. I head in their direction. It's about eight in the morning, and there are joggers and walkers out down by the lake edge with us, out for a casual bit of exercise on a nice Saturday morning, their faces registering an emotion partway between astonishment and pity upon hearing that our morning started twenty-four hours ago.

The closer I get to the lake, the bigger the houses. I reach the northern lakeshore. I pass huge mansions with metal gates and stone walls in front and surveillance cameras and signs that say PRIVATE PROPERTY—NO

TRESPASSING. Beyond the gates and warning signs, I see no evidence of human habitation. Beyond the mansions, I can see the giant azure mirror of the lake, shining in the dawn, circled by distant mountains. The mansions stand empty of their wealthy occupants. Asphalt smothers the earth. This is Washoe land. Before the Washoe, the land belonged to no one. Now the land lies slashed into little pieces, colonized by so-and-so as *mine*. At times like this, seeing civilization through high-country eyes, I understand why I used to need MDMA. My world felt split into bits back then. With the Eye of Cyclops, all I could see was the patch of reality in front of me. It was easy to forget how everything fit together: *even that it ever fit together at all*. Easy to forget that the way I thought of things, split into little fragments of reality, was just my way of seeing. When I was high and dancing, everything felt connected again and whole. The feeling sometimes lingered into the morning. But then it was gone. The *comedown*, as we ravers used to call it. And then I felt more disconnected and alone than ever, stuck in the empty mansion of my isolated mind. The feeling of bliss and unity on the dance floor was impossible to remember. Over time, this became its own sort of violence. But now I'm down by the lake, and I can still remember the feeling of running in the high country, seeing the horizon from far above.

VII

Saturn

The Field

The road by the lake leads to the highway, on the other side of which I can see an aid station. Tunnel Creek: mile 65. There's no sign of Miriam or my kids at Tunnel Creek. I get why. Miriam would have needed to drive from Brockway back to the rental house to get the kids and then schlep all the way to Tunnel Creek. I bet she's in bed. Good. I feel just about competent to take care of myself at this aid station. But only just about. I can feel the wheels of my thinking mind grinding just to manage even simple decisions. Volunteers are making pancakes on a little electric griddle. I have this sense of a gap between the drive to keep moving and the need to attend to a nonnegotiable but at this point fuzzy set of basic needs. To get the pancakes entails approaching a volunteer and saying, *Please can I have a pancake?* But hang on a second. What's this over here? Potato chips. Slices of watermelon. Would that make more sense first? What about changing shoes and socks, drinking . . . Is there anything else I'm supposed to do now? Is there an order? I stand by the table, waiting for my pancake. "What can I do you for, 108?" says one of the volunteers. "Please . . . can I have a pancake?" I manage to say. The volunteer puts the pancake mix on the griddle. I pick up a paper plate and load it with a quesadilla, some chips, and a couple of slices of melon. I pour a cup of coffee. I find a nearby camping chair. I sit down with my plate of food and my cup of coffee. I put the coffee cup in the little cup holder, put my plate of food on the chair, and then go look for my drop bag so I can change my socks. The bags are laid out on a tarp about a hundred feet down a slight slope closer to the road. I approach the pile. My eyes scan through the pile until I find the gray bag with my race number on it. I pick up the bag and go back to my chair. I put down the bag. I pick up my food plate and sit down. I put the food plate on the ground while I open the bag and hunt through it for a fresh pair of socks and a medical kit. I find what I'm looking for. I take off my shoes and socks. I wipe my feet down with alcohol wipes and dry them with baby powder. I wrap my blistered toes in medical tape. I scarf the pancake and chips and melon and quesadilla and chug the coffee and then I put on my fresh socks and heave myself from the chair before my legs seize up, and I yell, "108 heading out—thanks, everyone!" and I put on my earbuds, blaring house music, and march uphill in the morning light at the start of another massive climb back toward the high country. It's only nine in the morning and already it feels hot.

I'M HIKING UPHILL AROUND noon on a two-thousand-foot slog back to the high country. I'm facing east, with the sun right above me, baking down. Maybe it's not actually hotter than this time yesterday. But it sure feels that way. The experience of being outside in the elements has lost the smiley vacation feel of the early hours of the first climb yesterday and has turned into a feeling of exposure. The sun didn't change. I did. I'm tired and grumpy, and I have the start of this fuzzy-headed feeling that I know I need to do something about pronto. If I don't cool off soon, I'll end up like Boiling Man yesterday.

I spot a little creek. I drench my shirt and cap. The instant the cold mountain water hits my head, I feel better. As I hike up the trail, I can feel the water trickling down my neck. I eat a GU and pick up my pace.

The trail climbs about two thousand feet in around five miles on the way toward the Tahoe Rim Trail. A memory comes to me of a summer's day eleven years ago when I first ran there. My mind fills with images of the trail back then and the identical one now in front of me, two trails separated in clock time yet merging in my consciousness into one, as if each footfall on the ground propels me on a backward step in time.

It was my second attempt at a fifty-miler, on a hot day in early July about two years after I got out of the hospital. I stood among the runners in the cold dawn. Nobody asked me where I was from or what I did for a living. I'd left behind all the parts of me that weren't about getting my body up and down fifty miles of mountain trails. High school dropout or summa cum laude—it wasn't going to matter at ten thousand feet. It was chilly before the sun came up. I stood shivering next to a generator for warmth until the race director summoned us to the start line a little before 6 a.m. I heard the countdown from ten to zero and then I ran down the trail through a dark pine forest, the dusty ground illuminated in ghostly circles from a constellation of runners' headlamps, mirroring the stars, luminous above. The runners soon spread out and I had the trail to myself. By sunrise I had climbed to a high ridge from which I saw the lake thousands of feet below to the west, framed by a line of snow-flecked peaks. I followed the pink ribbons that marked the course every few hundred yards. I felt relieved from any worry about getting lost, from worry about anything. I knew where I was going, but I was in no rush to get there. Legs flowing, breathing easy, I traveled each mile in around ten or eleven minutes, a comfortable pace that felt just right—not too fast, but not slow either. With enough snacks and a nap now and then, I felt I could run like this across the whole world. I'd crossed a frontier into the unknown, aware that I was going to need to make do now with the body I had and not the fitter body I might have wanted. My life at home in San Francisco was in the past and the finish was far in the future, leaving the next few miles as the only reality.

Everywhere I looked there were beautiful lakes and mountains. A feeling came over me that I hadn't experienced in a long time, perhaps ever. I felt calm and alert and every sense dialed up a notch, the blue alpine sky and the smell of pine needles and sunscreen and the patch of trail right in front of me transforming with each step and the ease of my legs flowing and my chest rising and falling all merged and dancing together: it was bliss. I moved in this state of rapture longer than seemed legal. The Sierra Nevada is made from quadrillions of tons of granite, and my feeling of bliss felt equally massive, big enough to block out, at least for a while, all the anxious thoughts I'd been coping with for years, to provide a bodily answer to the ceaseless and seemingly unsolvable mysteries of my past that had put me in the hospital. As the hours passed and my legs tired from miles and miles of ascending and then descending steep mountain trails and the temperature climbed into the 70s and then into the 80s, I slowed and felt weak and a little light-headed, and I was suddenly aware of myself as isolated and seemingly close to total exhaustion, miles from help, and needing to stop soon while I still could voluntarily, rather than risk becoming a story in the local newspaper: ENGLISH MENTAL PATIENT SLAIN BY HIGH SIERRA HEATSTROKE, STUPIDITY. I followed the turns up the trail to a summit that I started to believe might actually be mythical, a symbolic rather than literal peak that would only come into existence if I believed in it. In response to the question *Why am I doing this?* I turned my mind toward each perception itself—a tree, a stone, the sun—as an answer in the form that Yoda might give to a young Jedi's inquiry about the nature of the Force: *Keep going on the trail you must.*

It was hard later to remember what I spent all those hours thinking about. But afterward, the long void of non-thinking felt like a kind of thought, but of a different quality than the thinking I did sitting down, although that difference eluded words. The thoughts I could recall were profundities like *Ow, that hurts*, when I stubbed my toe on a rock, or *Peanut-butter-and-jelly sandwiches are so much tastier when I'm hungry!* or *Wow, I'm tired*—when I was, uh, tired. But those thoughts arose within a space of non-thought that had tangible qualities, as if the trail at my feet and the trail of my mind were the same trail. The state had some similarities to the way I used to feel on psychedelic mushrooms, but it had a quieter, more sustainable feeling with fewer fireworks.

Hours passed. The bliss faded. I could remember the fun of the early miles in the way that I could remember that Ulaanbaatar was the capital of Mongolia. The end seemed to extend to an infinite horizon that I would never be able to reach. I screened the idea of finishing from my awareness, until its elimination even as a conceivable future intensified my distress. I climbed higher in the heat of the day, feeling more depleted and despairing with each step, my mind circling between two ideas of myself: finisher and loser. Around noon I reached a tent stationed at the halfway point, close to a road. I sat down in the shade, relieved to be done. I drank a cup of soda and ate. *I guess I've reached my limit. I guess this is all I've got. I was dumb to think a loser like me could do this.* What did I expect?

I started walking along the path that led to the road from where I hoped to hitch a ride. The road lay about a hundred feet up the path. Halfway to the road, the path joined another trail at a right angle. This other trail was marked with a ribbon that signified the start of the second half of the course. I stopped at the trail junction. I took another step forward. And another. A hundred feet along the trail, I started jogging. Half a mile farther, I was running again. A hundred yards below the summit, a boy scout ran to greet me. "Hello, Jason," he said, identifying me by the race number pinned to my shorts. "What do you need?" I needed more soda and cookies. I filled up on cookies and soda. I bent forward and touched my toes to ease the stiffness in my lower back and hamstrings. It was hard to get up again. "You got this," a volunteer said. "It's all downhill from here." The final seven miles would take another eternity, around an hour of thigh-punishing descent on a steep, rocky trail about a thousand feet down to the tree line and then several more hours winding down switchbacks through the forest to the finish at Spooner Lake, but knowing the end was at last close changed the sense of effort involved. After eight hours of sweat and hard effort, the fixtures of the past or uncertain future identity slipped away. At sunset I reached the highest point of the course, Snow Valley Peak, at an oxygen-starved altitude of 9,214 feet, from which a stunning panorama of lakes and mountains stretched seemingly to infinity in every direction. Before the final climb, I followed a trail through a meadow full of wildflowers. In his poem "A Great Wagon," Rumi wrote: "Out beyond ideas of wrong-doing and rightdoing, / there is a field. I'll meet you there."[13] I felt like Rumi's field was a physical one and I was in it.

I descended a rocky trail down to the tree line and into the forest, winding back and forth on a route through the trees toward the finish line, knowing Miriam and our baby daughter were waiting there, knowing that I was a father and a husband and an ultrarunner.

Something like this experience is the origin story of many an ultrarunner. You start out thinking a regular marathon sounds pretty far enough. There is an infamous low point around mile 18 when you get low on glycogen and feel like you can't keep going: the so-called wall. But eat something, drink something, and you keep going. You hit another wall, like I did at the midpoint of that fifty-mile race. You eat something, drink something. You keep going. You can keep on going on like that for a really, really long time.

Knowing this has an amazing effect on what seems possible not just in running but in the rest of your life. *I'm going to do it. I can do things.* It was a stunning revelation back then, the state I was in, to discover this. It's one thing to understand the arithmetic that a fifty-mile run is in reality a bunch of one-mile runs, stacked end to end, and another thing altogether to screen out all the messages that say that something like this is impossible. To shift your focus from *if* you can do it to *how.* I'd had that confidence, when I was little. But it had gotten lost along the way. To get it back I had needed proof of the most tangible kind there is: Moving. Going forward. Choosing a direction, and discovering that my choice meant something, so long as I kept on choosing it, one step at a time. Those steps took me to where I'm standing now, back on Snow Valley Peak, gazing at this incredible panorama of the lake thousands of feet below and the mountains in the distance. It's so majestic, there's a feeling of everything else falling away. No past. No future. Just the boundless *now.* Perhaps I've always been here.

Running from Birth and Death

I rode my bike up the hill from my apartment to the hospital. It was a steep climb that left me sweaty and panting by the time I got to the top. I locked my bike outside the hospital and went to a little coffee cart and bought a latte and a muffin. I went inside the hospital and took the elevator to the fourth floor. Down the corridor from the locked ward was a room with a circle of chairs. The official name was the Partial Hospitalization Program. Everyone called it Partial. The word felt apt. Everything in my life was partial. I was partially better, a partial human.

I sat down on one of the chairs and filled out my worksheet for the day, sipping my coffee. I wrote my name at the top and my number of days in Partial and what sort of mood I was in.

Day 11 . . . Glad to be here in Partial. I always feel a bit better after biking and drinking coffee. Still worried about Miriam and work. I don't think someone like me should be a parent. But I don't think I could handle being alone. I can't decide . . .

Around a quarter till nine the other patients drifted in and took their seats. Mike arrived. He was the director of the program. He was a clean-shaven man with neat dark hair and wearing slacks and a smart cotton sweater over a button-down shirt. He had kind eyes and the sort of New York accent that told the world he brooked no bullshit.

"The car exploded, and everyone burned to death," said a woman whose face was frozen like a ghost mask. Ten medications trials. "One word goes around in my head. From the autopsy. For the cause of death, I mean. *Incinerated.* The family was *incinerated*—I just can't get over how unbelievably horrific that sounds."

Mike invited each of us to speak. The group divided up in recognizable classes. Some of us were loudmouths and others were shy and still others altogether mute. Mike labored with great skill to cajole the loudmouths into listeners and persuade the mutes to speak. One time I was droning on about something or other when he interrupted me and asked me who I was talking to, and I said, "What are you talking about?" and he told me I was in my head, and I wondered where else I was supposed to be. I met a girl who looked nineteen or maybe twenty with bandages on both forearms from all the times she'd cut herself. I met a middle-aged man whose partner had jumped off the Golden Gate Bridge and who whenever he found himself within a five-mile radius of where his partner had died would drive there and walk to the spot on the bridge where his partner had climbed over the barrier and leapt into space, and he would look down at the dark water hundreds of feet below and contemplate whether to join him. He couldn't help it, he said, going back there. It was the same with almost everything he did, he said. "Totally OCD." He would get into something, and the next thing he knew, it had taken over his life. In a previous lifetime, before his boyfriend died, he was an endurance athlete. He raced Ironman triathlons and had spreadsheets tracking every mile and workout and his maximum aerobic capacity measured in cubic milliliters of oxygen. Then he gave all that up and got into coffee. He soon ramped up to twenty-five cups every day. I met a large man who had recently declared bankruptcy and who talked a lot more than the rest of us combined. I thought he was totally full of himself until one time I was talking about how terrified I was of becoming a father because babies need love and I didn't have any love to give, and he said, "When that baby comes out, something happens—soon as you see it, you'll feel love, I guarantee it."

After group, Mike or one of his colleagues assigned us some homework. The curriculum diverged from the list of ancient Greek verbs and chemical formulae and poetry quotations I had been required to memorize at King Edward's and at college in England. It involved lessons about how to live. Apparently it was possible to feel horrible and think, *Fuck this. I'm leaving the country or jumping in front of a train*, but without actually doing either of those things. Suppose you hate the color purple, said the psychologist in the video we watched. Her name was Marsha Linehan. Your house is being painted. You come home—guess what color it is. But what are you going to do? Now you have a purple house. Suck it up, buttercup. Accept it. That doesn't mean you have to like it. But there it was. You remember your old house, before it was purple. You picture the new house, the way you wanted it to be. But no amount of remembering or wishing would ever turn the ruined house in the present into the nonexistent house you yearned to live in.

SATURN IS THE GOD of time. I once saw an article in a running magazine that defined a speedy so-and-so's accomplishments with the statement that he "owned" a certain time in the marathon. It struck me as an odd expression. A person can own many things, but time is not among them. Even Bezos couldn't buy it. Nobody owns time—time owns us. It would be hard to imagine colonizing something so elusive to articulation. As Saint Augustine wrote in his *Confessions*: "What, then, is time? If no one asks me, I know; if I wish to explain to him who asks, I know not."

Aristotle said he knew. For Aristotle, time was change. You see green leaves go brown in the autumn and infer that time has passed. But what is it in this that has passed? And if time is change, then does time itself change, or is time timeless? Early Christian writers conceived of a timeless order independent of change: the Kingdom of God. The Christian notion of a timeless order was the philosophical background that inspired Isaac Newton's definition of time in the 1600s as an absolute uniform dimension, divisible in linear terms like space. For Newton, time was Out There: the past had a street address. But then along came Einstein, who proved that time isn't absolute—and neither, indeed, is space. Both are relative to the position of an observer. More recent cosmology suggests that the kind of time we talk about when we split things up into past, present, and future bears no relation at all to the reality of the universe. Time—of the subjective passing variety—doesn't match what's really Out There. Even a moment of the most cursory introspection illuminates the truth that no entity resembling absolute time exists in our *experience* either.

At the level of ultimate cosmic reality, then, time might be an illusion. But it is an enduring one. In almost all societies throughout history, humanity has understood time in a tripartite division between past, present, and future. We talk about time in terms of space. The past is *behind* us. The future is *ahead*. Under ordinary circumstances, that's how it feels. Memories of events that occurred a long time ago feel like they've receded to a vanishing point in the rearview mirror of the mind.

But trauma sabotages the normal experience of a moment's gradual recession into what feels *past*. Evolution has hardwired the brain and nervous system to privilege the mechanisms that enable us to survive threats that either are happening in the immediate present or are imminent. The unconscious tells the traumatized person: *Get ready. The disaster might happen again. It might still be happening.* If the trauma feels behind us at all, it's lurking right over our shoulder, ready to pounce. When the normal, neat division of past, present, and future gets messed with like this, what's past can feel like it's present, and feelings connected to recent events can retroactively shape the recollection of earlier ones. Trauma sends shock waves back into the remembered past. Life collapses into a single ongoing emergency: the time it's always been.

..

I drove down the snowy road. I couldn't see the white lines on the tarmac. It was hard to know where I was supposed to go. "You're driving on the wrong side," said Sebastian. I was glad he had come to visit. I could always count on Sebastian. A ski trip had been Sebastian's idea. Or maybe it was Mike's. "If he gets stuck in his head, throw him in the snow," Mike had said. We had driven to Lake Tahoe and checked into a motel. The weather was so bad we couldn't see the lake or the mountains surrounding it. Everything was snowy and misty.

When we got up that morning, I went to the closet to grab the ski clothes I'd dumped in a pile on the floor on one side. I looked at Sebastian's clothes, which he'd hung in neat rows on the other side.

My thoughts drifted to a family ski trip decades earlier. In my mind's eye, I could recall the moment when a colossal landscape loomed into view, resplendent in the dawn sun, of snowy mountains extending in every direction to a far horizon. None of us, except Sebastian—who had taken lessons on a dry slope—had put on skis before, and we struggled to put our boots into the ski bindings. I remembered becoming sweaty and overheated with the effort while wearing ski clothes in the mild sunny weather, and an irritable exchange of words then occurring—I forget the details—between my mother and me. "Right, that's it," she said. "No more skiing." It was incomprehensible: We'd bought ski clothes, flown from Heathrow to Germany, driven by bus through a blizzard to the Austrian Alps, rented skis and boots, gotten weeklong lift passes and ski lessons—it must have cost thousands—but dawn on day one and Mum was calling the whole thing off?

Her decision was incontestable. I appealed to Dad—any sane person would surely recognize the folly of squandering such a precious chance in the mountains—but he appeared powerless to countermand or even question her. I couldn't remember how we filled the empty days that followed. I could remember gazing at the mountains and daydreaming of an older version of myself holding hands with my imaginary girlfriend, the two of us frolicking in the snow like George Michael and the pretty girl in the "Last Christmas" video. *Tell me, baby, do you recognize me? Well, it's been a year, it doesn't surprise me . . ."* Sebastian and I spent some time admiring ski equipment in the village shop windows and chatting about which brand looked the coolest, Atomic or Rossignol or Dynastar. Then we followed Mum and Dad into a fancy clothing store, where Sebastian and I were allowed to pick something expensive—designer jeans, perhaps—as if we were clinging to the pretense of a family enjoying a holiday together, engaged in a shopping trip after a day on the slopes. As the week's end drew near, my dismay drifted into resignation. On New Year's Eve my mother drank a whole bottle of wine at dinner, and I was woken later that night by the sound of her vomiting, and 1987 began with the sight of Mum asleep on the bathroom floor, curled around the toilet. Later that morning I saw a poster in the village advertising a pig-catching competition and its presumed favorite, a champion in prior years—a pig called Clifford Oily—and a picture of Clifford and some burly men in lederhosen attempting to catch him formed in my mind with such vivid detail that as I recalled that champion pig in Austria standing in a Tahoe motel room decades later, I wasn't sure if the pig-catching competition had existed in reality or only my imagination, so when I remembered the Austrian Alps, I couldn't help but picture greased pigs slipping through the hands of men tumbling over in the snow in an effort to capture them, and the comfort I felt in mentally conjuring this absurd scene while Sebastian and my father and I followed our mother into the frozen darkness.

Sebastian and I reached the ski slopes. Ahead of us was the task of renting skis and boots and poles and buying lift tickets and going to the bathroom and getting to the lift and taking it to the top of the mountain. Was it tickets first and skis second, or bathroom, skis, tickets? . . . I might as well have been a medieval farmer made to take a college math exam. "I can't remember the order," I said. "Do we get the skis or . . ." I couldn't finish the sentence. "Let's get the tickets, then the skis and boots," said Sebastian. *Who is this Einstein?*

We got up the mountain. I turned my skis to face downhill. I gathered speed. I lost control, and as I tumbled into the deep, powdery snow, my skis detached from their bindings. "Need any help?" said Sebastian. "No," I said. I put my skis back on and pushed off with my poles, and soon I was flying downhill with the icy wind in my face. *I can remember this used to be fun. But now I can't feel anything. Nothing at all. Something must really have broken inside of me. Now I'm thinking again. Stop it. Don't think. Don't think about how if you feel numb here, you'll feel numb everywhere. Stop it. . . . That was a thought. The thought about thinking that you're not supposed to be thinking about how you're thinking how you're not supposed to be thinking.*

That night we went to the movies. In the middle of some action flick in which the hero was dying, my head spun into a loop about which was better, staying alive in my horrible state or not being here anymore, until the thoughts were so loud in my head I couldn't bear the noise and I ran out of the movie and went to watch another one on the next screen over in the multiplex, something schmaltzy with violin music, but then it got to this part with a little baby, and seeing the baby, my head spun in a different loop about being a dad and how impossible that was for a broken man like me, so I ran out of that movie too and into the one on the other side of the corridor, and then back and forth, between every screen in the theater, but all of the movies were the same: there was no running away from birth and death.

··

I didn't know what to expect from the meeting with my father. I didn't know why I had asked for it. The words had just tumbled out of my mouth one morning after group. "My father's in town—would you like to meet him?" After he heard the story from Miriam about the knife and the pills and the bloody wound on my leg, it took him a couple of weeks to get on a plane to California. Miriam was less than pleased. "There's no way I can come now," Dad had apparently told her. "I'd be useless." I understood. *Yeah, that's right, you'd be useless.* I couldn't imagine him being useful. When he did show up, Miriam didn't bend over backward to disguise her displeasure. "It must remind him of what he went through when he was my age, back in Cannon

Road," I said. Miriam would have none of it. "He's your father! He's supposed to be here!"

Dad strolled into Mike's office and sat down. Mike shook his hand. Dad told him about the hard times in Cannon Road and how they all began, he now realized, when Granddad died and Gran sold the house by the mountain and he lost any semblance of connection to his childhood home in Ireland, like a tree uprooted from the particular soil that had nourished it and shoved into the ground somewhere far away. Perhaps this was my problem too, said Dad, uprooting myself from England and the entire life I had known.

Mike nodded and took notes and then asked me what I thought of Dad's interesting idea, and I said, "The truth is, Mike, I'm feeling very numb at the moment," and at once I saw a look of intense concern form on Mike's face. "I'm sending you back to the unit," he said. "What?" I said. Dad looked stunned. "You've been here in Partial for weeks. Then you ask for this very impromptu meeting with your father. Then you talk about feeling numb. It's a communication. You're telling me you're planning to kill yourself. Maybe you can't say it straight. But that's the message you're giving me, even if you're not aware of it."

I spent the weekend back in the inpatient unit. At Mike's prompting, I had a consultation for ECT. The ECT doctor was a man who reportedly specialized in the procedure and had administered it to hundreds of patients and knew everything there was to know about it. His manner was courteous. I experienced no explicit coercion from him. Yet I had the impression he was a person with a narrow or perhaps exclusive focus on his chosen skill, and that having entered this psychiatric barbershop, so to speak, I could expect to leave with a head shock. "You will be sedated," he said. "We'll put electrodes on your head. A low-voltage current goes into your brain. We induce a little seizure. It's very low risk. You might lose your memories of the time just before the procedure. But you might also feel less depressed."

I asked for a second opinion. Sometime later I found myself sitting on the blacktop with a senior psychiatrist. He was an older man in spectacles with a full professorship. He asked me to tell him the history of my illness from as early as I could remember. I spoke for a long time. He listened. I could sense him listening to every word I said and absorbing every detail with great caring and acuity. "It doesn't sound like you have the kind of depression that would *necessarily* be helped by ECT," he said. In the end, I didn't go through with the procedure. If I lost my memories, who would I be?

The Lost Men

The two-thousand-foot descent from Snow Valley Peak follows a rocky trail down to the tree line that then winds through the forest to the next aid station near the highway. It's around four in the afternoon on Saturday and still very warm. When I reach the aid station, I see a bunch of runners lying out on the ground, getting some kip. Man, it would feel good to join them. After almost a second full day on my feet, I'm feeling exhausted and woozy from all the uphill marching and high mountain sun. But if I lie down, I'm not sure when I'll manage to get up again. I guess I'll see how I feel after I've filled up on food and fluids. I sit down with a big cup of soda with ice and a plate of food. I sip the soda. *Yum.* There probably isn't a single thing in the world that would taste any better right now than these twelve ounces of ice-cold sugar water.

I drain the soda and wolf down a couple of quesadillas and some salty chips and boiled potatoes and a peanut-butter-and-jelly sandwich, then I get up, fill one of my bottles with more cold soda and the other with electrolyte drink, then down some of the electrolyte drink, drench my neck and head in cold water, and march out of said station toward the trailhead and back up the mountain, heading south in the still-fierce heat of late afternoon.

I'M ALMOST HALFWAY AROUND the lake now. Quite a thought. I merge into the rhythm of uphill hiking as the sun sinks lower toward the horizon. Looking across the lake from its eastern side, I can see the mountains in the west where my run began. I can remember looking across the water from Homewood, a day and a half ago, toward the peaks where I am running now. The background has become the foreground;

the future has become present. I feel myself merge with the pink and gold radiance of the evening, with the rhythm of my march up the mountain, while the light begins to fade.

THE TRAIL'S BEEN HEADING downhill in the dark for much longer than seems fair or reasonable. I'm not blaming the mountains for being high or the lake for being far away. But a hundred miles and thirty-six hours in and just this sort of dreamy illogic is getting harder to resist. Once in a while I can see what looks like a ski lodge, lit up in multicolored lights like a fairy-tale castle, a long, long way down by the lake. What I can remember of the course profile for this section is that it's basically up, then down—like this: ∧. I'm on the downward slope of that pyramid. So I'm assuming the fairy castle is Heavenly Ski Resort: mile 102. Halfway. Nap time. Miriam will be there. My friends Emily and her husband, Andrew, will be there. Miriam and Andrew will tuck me in and help me go night-night. Then Emily will join me running for the next eighty miles. *Get to Heavenly. Get to Miriam and Andrew and Emily and all the friendly, generous people. Then you can rest. Heaven knows you deserve it.*

The castle disappears. All I can see is the little path of steep trail below me and the dark forest. *Really? Screw you too, Mountain—I never liked you anyway.* Down, down, down, and now I'm at the bottom of the mountain. No sign of the castle. I remember it being over to my right. But now the trail's heading left. Away from the lake. Away from the castle. The trail's been going this way and that, higgledy-piggledy—surely any minute now it will cut back right again. Back to the lake. Back to the castle. But that's not what happens. I'm heading even farther from the lake *and then uphill again. What? Am I lost?* No, I see a course marker. This has to be the right way. Only it feels so wrong. In theory, I could stop. I could look at the map, try to figure out where I am. But I'm so very tired. I don't have it in me. *Please just put me to bed, Mountain. I've been such a good boy. Haven't I, Mountain? Please take me to the castle.*

The trail heads deeper into the trees. I come across a little group of runners. Three men. "Where's Heavenly?" I say. "Are we off course?" "Who the hell knows. GPS says no. But this makes no sense. We should be there now." I should be there now. And yet we are not. We are the Lost Men, abandoned in the darkness, forever trudging up an endless hill and never getting home. *Mountain has decided.* We fall into single file as the trail heads up steep switchbacks that go on and on and on.

"WHEN WAS THE LAST time anyone saw a course marker?" I say. Silence. All I want right now is to be lying down. *Please make this stop.* One of the Lost Men says his GPS has us at 104 miles. This can't be right. A sort of angst starts gnawing at me. If we're really off course, there's no telling how much longer it'll take to find our way back on course again—but if this is really where I'm meant to be right now, well, then, I don't like it. Could this uphill be a little blip on the downhill slope of the ∧? But it goes on so long, that just doesn't seem credible.

At the side of the trail I see an extremely old man. His head is drooping forward, in a gesture of defeat. *What's this old man doing out here all by himself in the forest? Wait, that's impossible.* The old man turns into a burned-out pine tree. My mind is playing tricks on me. I see an infinity of trees and darkness. I contemplate the thought that one day all the stars will burn out and all the light will go out in the universe.

"Seriously, when was the last time anyone saw a course marker?" I say. Silence from the Lost Men.

"How far have we gone?" I say.

"About 103," says one of the Lost.

"About 106," says another.

Am I ever getting out of here?

STOP. THINK. I REMEMBER something. In my pocket I have a little piece of laminated paper illustrating the sawtooth profile of the course. I don't need to keep marching onward through the dark in despair. I need to stop. Think. Get my bearings. Make a plan. If I really am lost, so be it. I'll deal with it. Better to know you're lost and change course back in the right direction than keep heading in the wrong direction and ignoring the evidence of your eyes, trying to kid yourself you're not really lost.

One time I did just that in the middle of the night about halfway through a 120-mile run in the mountains of British Columbia. I hadn't seen a single soul in eons. In the pre-race meeting the day before, the race director said, "If you don't see a course marker after you've gone a mile, assume you've gone off course, and turn around." There were supposed to be course markers every half-mile. I hadn't seen one in I didn't know how long. I was in a zombie state, marching ahead, oblivious to logic and the empty fire road that stretched farther into nowhere without the slightest trace of a course marking or another runner for a great long while. But by then I had invested such an effort down this dark, empty path, it felt like such a waste to give up on it, especially since I had not bothered to check my watch for some indeterminate passage of time and felt my mind drift into a state where that indeterminate stretch of time could have been five minutes as easily as fifty. I kept going. In this fatigue-induced state—a kind of regression into the delusions of magical omnipotence that characterize the minds of very young children—it then occurred to me that if there was any justice in the universe the course markers surely ought to appear soon enough simply because I had struggled so hard in the direction where in good faith I had imagined their existence. Yet as the trail wound farther into the darkness, the re-alization came to me that I was lost, and I turned back and ran the five miles I'd gone off course.

I made that mistake in British Columbia only a couple of years ago. I have no desire to repeat it. So I do stop and look at the course profile. I get my bearings right away. The course is just a single long descent to Heavenly. My memory had failed me. What I see now isn't as simple as the up-down picture I have had in my mind. It's more like this: ∧∧. At the top of the second smaller pyramid there's a red dot, marking the aid station. Okay, now this makes sense: I'm done with the first big pyramid, and I'm somewhere on the upward slope of the second, smaller one. *What a dumb way to spend my time. Who put that extra mountain there? Ri-dic-u-lous. I should quit. That'll show 'em! Stop whining. You're frickin' exhausted is all. Get to Heavenly. It can't be more than twenty minutes max from here. Miriam will be there. Emily and Andrew will be there. Then you'll sit down. Soak your feet in ice water. Eat. And then you'll get some kip. You'll head out with Emily into a new day. Everyone's done so much to help you. You absolutely cannot quit. Not yet, anyway . . .*

THE TRAIL LEADS DOWN to the ski lodge, where I can see Miriam bundled up in warm clothes. There's a man standing next to her whom I don't recognize. "What do you need?" he says. This man is here to help me, it seems. What kindness exists in the universe: it is a marvel.

I sit down. Miriam wraps a sleeping bag around me. Kindness asks me again what I might need. "Food," I say. He lists the foods available. Soup is among them. "Soup," I say. "Can I get you anything else?" says Kindness, the Knower of Names. "Cold water for my feet," I say. Kindness is gone, then reappears, bearing a cold chest filled with water. "Thank you," I tell Kindness, the Granter of Wishes.

I take off my shoes and socks. I put my feet into the water. The cold soothes their painful swelling. I drink my soup.

Miriam and Kindness help me stand. I hobble inside the lodge to a large dining room that has been converted into a makeshift sleeping area. The whole room is full of exhausted runners, lying on the floor in sleeping bags. I can see their weary faces, hear the silence of the nighttime hours punctured by a chorus of moans and farts and snores. I lie down among them, my legs propped up on a chair, feeling my calf and thigh muscles stiffen and throb with pain, and join the chorus of moans.

"When would you like me to wake you?" says Kindness, looming above me now from my position laid out flat on an inflatable mattress on the floor. "Two hours," I say. In the light of the ski lodge interior, the face of Kindness becomes visible. It's Andrew. In my exhausted state, I hadn't recognized him. I drift into the twilight between dreams and waking, and soon I am running in the dream forest, the convergence of the remembered trail and the paths that lead inward to everything imaginable. I watch the dream leaves dance in an imaginary wind and I become them.

VIII

Uranus

The Horizon

I wake after two hours of restless sleep. My body is as stiff as a board. It's difficult to stand. I hobble downstairs on swollen, blistered feet to the communal bathroom. I'm moving really slowly. My mind's not doing much better. It's hard to think straight. *Go to the bathroom . . . Stretch . . . Yes, that's the right order . . .*

Several runners are seated on chairs at the foot of the stairs, outside the bathroom, getting ready to head back out on the trail. Their faces have the crumpled and shattered look of souls drained into states of utter depletion, persevering on quests of mysterious purpose, like weary ghosts in exile from the world they once knew, someplace now faded and almost forgotten.

I go into the bathroom to splash some water on my face and clean my teeth. I see the man in the mirror: me. *English male, disheveled . . .* I've seen and thought and felt more in the past two days than the previous forty years. But there's one thing I haven't seen, because it's invisible: *Me.* When I look in the mirror, my perspective flips from inside looking out to outside looking in, from I to me, between the world as it shows up in my awareness and the way I show up to others. They're so unlike each other, this mirror me and I, it's almost hard to believe we're the same person.

I leave the bathroom. Andrew is in the lobby outside with Emily. She's in her running clothes, after a few hours of sleep in her car, ready to go now. Andrew hands me a plate of food. It's hard to get the food down. I have no sensation of hunger, my lips are chapped and dry from two days in the mountain sun, and for some reason my tongue hurts.

I take off my socks to inspect my foot damage. There are several blisters between the toes on both feet. I put some antibiotic cream on the blisters and wrap my toes with medical tape. I put my socks back on. I crouch on my hands and knees to do some yoga stretches to loosen up my shoulders, neck, legs, and back. Then I sit down, drink a cup of coffee, and put on a change of shoes.

"Ready?" says Emily. I nod yes. I feel more awake now, but not by much. I've slept four hours in the past forty-four. My head is fuzzy. I look at my watch. It's around half past four in the morning. Between getting up and being ready to go, it's been more than an hour.

I'm glad I took the time.

I grab my poles and follow Emily out of the lodge into the cold early morning air. As I get into a good hiking rhythm behind Emily, my mind starts clearing up and my legs feel more limber.

"Water," says Emily.

I take a sip. "Thanks," I say. I'm grateful for the reminder to stay hydrated. I'm 110 miles in. You run 50 miles on your own brain. Past that point, when the thinking mind turns off, you need a second brain, someone still awake and compos mentis who can do the thinking for you: a pacer, as they're called. He or she might help set your physical pace, but for the most part their role is to remember and plan and reason when your brain can no longer perform those functions. Maybe you should drink something. Maybe you should eat something. Keep going, and you'll get there in the end. Everyone knows that. In normal circumstances, yes. But not after you've run 110 miles. In my current state, the only thing I can remember is the need to keep moving. So it's good I have Emily with me. As far as second brains go, I couldn't hope for a better one.

The trail gains two thousand feet from Heavenly to Armstrong Pass. The rising sun in a cloudless azure sky casts the arid sand pyramid of Freel Peak above us in a golden aura. At close to ten thousand feet, the pass is the highest point of the course. The air is thinner at that altitude. I feel light-headed. The long, breathless slog uphill is worth it for the view. In the early morning light in the pure high-mountain air, every single visible thing, every tree and creek and peak and bird and flower, shines with a crystal luminosity. Nothing could have such crisp edges, such a shimmer of living radiance both outside and within. It is perfect. Complete. Unsurpassable.

We stand in the morning light, gazing across at the vast green wilderness and at the mountains far away.

WE ALL START OUT with the same view, the inside of a womb. But we're each born into a different world. At first, it's a blur: we can see just far enough to glimpse Mom's or Dad's face. Our eyes flicker back and forth, the quick motions called saccades, shooting signals from the optic nerves to the brain, where over time the dance of light forms into names of things, a smile or a frown, a shoe or a spoon, and we learn that day turns into night and a leaf blows away but some things persist. Over time, we explore the terrain that stretches beyond the cradle, our house and neighborhood to the planet beyond. We find out that there are two ways of looking at things: the up-close-and-personal world of our own joys and worries and the wider world that extends to the Arctic pole and the troposphere and from there to Uranus. The ancient Greeks thought of Uranus as the god of the sky.

The brain has separate processes for those two distinct ways of seeing. Look at your hand and it is a single thing that belongs to you. The brain sends signals from sound and sight and touch to the top front layer of your brain. This allows you to shift your attention quickly to anything to the left or right, up or down. By the time the signals reach the regions of your brain that support so-called focal attention, they also have stimulated regions connected to memory and emotion and what happens to you and what is yours.

But look at the horizon from a high place or stare into the night sky and it's not about you. Another neural pathway starts at the back of the brain and runs forward to the temporal and frontal lobes and supports a wider view: global attention. This is the way you see how objects stand in relation to one another rather than to yourself. Global attention enables you to see things beyond what's you and yours, independently of your needs or their capacity to hurt or help you.

When you can picture the world beyond the up-close version, shifting to a broader, global, or even cosmic perspective, new possibilities come into view. When our evolutionary ancestors progressed from crouching to walking on two legs, they could see farther. They also started to see themselves: the cave paintings of Lascaux depict hunting but also the Paleolithic mind's emergent self-awareness. To astronauts viewing Earth from hundreds of miles above in space, the atmosphere looks like a razor-thin layer, and they are often overwhelmed by a phenomenon known as the overview effect, a poignant awareness of the planet as a single interconnected system. They realize that the sky must be protected so it will exist for future generations, that from the perspective of Earth's orbit national boundaries are fictions, and that as living beings we share a single home.

The high country extends beyond the mountains. It's not so much a physical place as a way of being. It's looking up into the night sky and wondering. It's Stephen Hawking imagining black holes. It's the view from the high country both literal and symbolic: the Tibetan plateau viewed from the summit of K2 and the equitable society conceived in the mountaintop vision of Martin Luther King Jr. It's the best of who we are and what we might become.

Everyone should see the horizon from a hill. Down below you see someplace you know from ground level. You spot somewhere else familiar. Then you see how the two places stand in relation to each other, the trails that link them together. The links have always been there. But down on the ground you couldn't see them. Maybe down on the ground, the other side of town seemed like a different reality.

Lines

Days turned into weeks. The feeling of sitting after the hard effort on the bike with the coffee and muffin appeared every morning for about ten minutes and then was gone, leaving in its wake the same old ache and fear and looping thoughts. *Nothing has changed. I still can't think straight.*

One morning I was sitting in group, thinking, when everything froze. Time stopped. I stopped. Everything appeared with the machinelike quality of a world where there had never been any such thing as a human mind, a world where nothing was recognizable or had a name, a world where nothing felt like anything at all because there was nobody left to feel it. Not chairs but hard, cold squares of matter. No people on the chairs but round lumps atop the square ones. *This is existence. It has always been this way.* Fear took hold of me. *What happened? Who am I? What am I?* Fear flipped into terror. *What if I'm stuck like this? I would rather be dead. This is much worse than death, whatever this is. Being frozen. Hell. I must be in hell. Help. Oh God, please help . . .*

The following series of realizations then took shape in my shattered consciousness: *I'm thinking things. Seeing people and chairs and the gray light through the windows. Eyes that see things and ears that hear them. I am me, and all of this out there is not-me . . .*

A gap had opened up between perceptions and perceiver that restored me to a recognition of me sitting there, feeling scared, eyes darting around the room, until my gaze met Mike's and I understood that he had seen me. I went to talk to him after group. I tried to put my horrific experience into words.

"It's called depersonalization," he said in a calm and gentle tone. "It happens. It's nothing to get too worried about."

"But what if it happens again?" I said.

"Maybe it will. Maybe it won't. You'll be okay."

"How do you know?" I cried.

"Because I have faith in you."

"I don't see how that's possible," I said, "if I don't have faith in myself."

"I know you don't," he said. "And that's why I have faith in you. I'm going to hold the faith for you."

He was looking right at me. I couldn't remember anyone ever looking at me like that, the way his eyes really saw me. I couldn't remember anyone ever talking to me like that, the way his voice was so soft and gentle. *You understand what I'm going through, even though I don't. You can see a path out of this darkness, even if I can't. You're not going to leave me alone here, crying in the dark. You've been here before. You know the way out.*

Day 40. Wish I could stay in Partial forever. Afraid to go back to work.

I walked into the office building. *I might as well be wearing a sign on my head saying* MENTAL PATIENT, I thought. When Mike and the other therapists had mentioned the prospect of my eventual return to work, I was terrified. Returning to my isolated office cubicle had been unimaginable. I didn't think I would be able to write grants in my disabled state of mind, and I worried about the way people would look at me. *Everyone will know where I've been all this time. I won't be me anymore. I'll be that guy who lost it and went to the psych ward. The mental patient.*

"Don't think of going back as all-or-nothing," Mike had said. "We'll take it one day at a time." My return to work would involve a gradual transition, he had explained. In the first couple of weeks I would go to the office for just a single day per week. Being there might bring up difficult thoughts and feelings, he said. But I could bring those thoughts and feelings back to Partial. When I was ready, I would spend two days per week at work, then three, then four, and I would only go back to a full five-day week when I was ready.

I walked upstairs to the second floor of the building. I saw Jessica, the receptionist. *Uh-oh.* "Jason!" she said with a big smile on her face.

I approached my cubicle. A middle-aged woman in the adjacent cubicle spotted me as I neared my desk. Her name was Moira. "Welcome back, Jason," she said, looking straight into my eyes and opening her arms, in the offer of a hug. "It's so great to see you."

So great to see me? What? Moira had always struck me as a down-to-earth sort of person. But in the three years I'd worked for the organization I could count the conversations we'd had on the fingers of one hand. I was surprised she'd even noticed that I'd been gone.

OH, THE HORROR OF another day. I wished I could go back to sleep. I wished I could close my eyes and never wake up again. I lay in bed, waiting for the ache of living to subside, waiting for the despair and dread and runaway thinking to ease, waiting to bear the idea of pulling back the covers and climbing out of bed, waiting for the vision of a tolerable future, waiting for hope to begin. I thought about suicide all the time. I went online and ordered a guidebook on how to do it. I forget the author and the title. But I will never forget something the author said, in between the passages outlining the pros and cons of the various standard methods: "For all I know, this might be the last book you'll ever read. Please consider carefully whether you really want to do this." There was something about the tone of that *you*: I could feel the presence of another human being, reaching across the chasm between us. I felt like he was talking to me. He wanted the best for me. He didn't want me to die. He respected me enough to talk about this horrible thing, feeling so terrible I might need to kill myself, without getting mad at me or crying. He reminded me of Mike.

I wished I could take up permanent residence in Partial. I felt safer there. But following the plan I had worked out with Mike, I was committed to a gradual transition back to work. I had to learn to cope with the world outside the hospital. I had to learn how to tolerate the ache that took hold of me from the very first moment I woke in the morning until I took my pills last thing at night and fell asleep. That was one thing I liked: the way those pills felt. There was this nice little reprieve, a few minutes after I took the pills, when the drugs started kicking in, when the ache faded away and left a calm feeling. In the hospital, Mike had told me to write down, every day, three things I was grateful for. Ideally, he said, it should be three different things each time. But if I couldn't think of new things, that was okay. I could write the same things each time, so long as I was really grateful for them. "But what if I can't think of three things?" I said. "What if I can't think of even one?" "Do your best," he said. So I wrote down "my pills." I was grateful for that brief, calm feeling, the moment between swallowing the pills and losing consciousness. I wished it would last longer. I wished I could lie there with my head on the pillow and my eyes closed, without the ache but still awake, forever. Sometimes as I lay there with the calm feeling I would also feel Miriam's finger tracing little circles on my arm. It felt nice. So the second thing I was grateful for was Miriam stroking my arm. The third thing was chocolate. I'd never lost my appetite. Some of the pills made me feel hungry all the time. I could eat and eat and eat but not feel full. I devoured fistfuls of candy. Chocolate, pills, and Miriam's finger: those were my only favorite things. The rest of the time, I tried to cope with the ache. Unless I was eating sweets or lying down in bed after the pills kicked in, or feeling Miriam's finger, or sleeping, I was hurting. I wasn't sure how much longer I could handle it.

My first assignment back at work was the kind of task that a functional twelve-year-old could have done. The task in question involved reorganizing text documents in the folder architecture of my desktop hard drive. Review all the old grant files on the hard drive, Glenda said. Sort the files into topics. Make one folder per topic. If there are lots of files on one topic, sort them into categories, and make subfolders. But my thoughts refused to sort themselves into subfolders. Marooned inside my cubicle walls, I felt a strange restlessness. It was less the physical desire to flee the building than a mental discomfort with every single instant of experience, the need for each present moment to vanish and turn into the past. *Make this now go away . . . and this now . . . and this now . . .* I had a bizarre perception of time moving too slowly, and the weird anxiety that without my conscious willing this temporal momentum into being, time might stop and freeze me in an eternal now.

Folders and subfolders . . . categories and topics . . . It was hard to tolerate being alone with my own mind. My mind was dangerous: it had tried to kill me. I yearned for contact with anything outside it, no matter how mundane or trivial. I would open my email inbox and read every new message, even junk mail and spam. "Esteemed friend, Greetings from Lagos—I have recently come into possession of one hundred million dollars." What comfort I felt in the awareness of another human mind, trying to reach mine, even if only in an attempt to deceive me. I discovered an underground office subculture of time-wasting resistance expressed through the exchange of winking emoticons and silly chats on instant messenger. What relief I felt in joining this kind of talk, which was never about anything so much as the wish for talk itself, the feeling in each electronic ping announcing the arrival of a new IM of a fellow human soul in the universe and the assurance that I still existed in the minds of others and they in mine.

Between acknowledging every smiley face emoji and Nigerian email scam, my progress on the subfolders was halting. I showed Glenda what I had done. She provided further instructions. I returned to my cubicle. I tried again. This cycle repeated itself. With an audible sigh of a busy person at the end of her patience, Glenda then narrated the exact sequence of computer keystrokes required to assemble the folder hierarchy. I wrote the instructions down. I returned to Dr. Jensen. He prescribed a high dose of Effexor, an antidepressant whose mechanism of action combines the effects of serotonin and norepinephrine reuptake inhibitors, as well as Abilify, an antipsychotic medication often used as an augmentation strategy for treatment-resistant depression. Soon after I took those drugs in combination, I felt a subtle shift in the void that had engulfed me. It is hard to express this shift in language. It was like some sort of restoration of an inner brightness. As spring turned into summer, my suicidal thoughts began to fade. But they did not disappear. The idea of death by suicide still loomed in my thoughts as a sort of psychic escape hatch, a horrific yet necessary exit strategy from the pain of staying alive if living hurt too much.

One day I saw a trailer for the forthcoming remake of *The War of the Worlds*. *How exciting that looks!* I thought. *I should definitely see it before I kill myself.* It occurred to me that a person who really wants to die doesn't make a plan to see a movie.

Still, the ache of depression did not subside. I didn't feel quite so bad—but neither did I ever really feel good. I went back to the ocean. The freezing-cold water took the ache away. When I rode a wave, I felt a little spike of euphoria that made a whoop sound come out of me. But I was a terrible surfer: if I even got up on a single wave, I was lucky. And after I was dry and warm and back at work, there was the ache again, as bad as ever. "I want you to whoop at work," Mike had said. What a joke. *Fuck yeah, today I'm writing grants!* When the world ended and aliens wrote the history of Earth, I bet they wouldn't find a single human who'd ever said those words. Whoop at work? If I could have made a sound, it would have been a whimper like a sick dog in a cage. So I sat in my cubicle, typing nonsense in IM, eating candy.

I MADE EYE CONTACT with a young man in a hoodie. "Sorry we crashed your party, man," he said. "My friends and I were talking, and we decided we ought to try and make it up to you. We came up with a proposal." In his pocket the man had a small bag of what back in England I used to know as Charlie: cocaine. "I accept your proposal," I said. I led him to the bathroom. He poured out the cocaine and chopped it into lines with a credit card. I snorted a line. A sphere of euphoric focus formed around me. *Hello, Charlie*, I said. *Hello, little one*, said Charlie.

If I could have frozen the feeling of being held by Charlie until the end of time, I would have done so. Charlie and I were old friends— lovers, even. One summer in the late '90s, a couple of years before I met Miriam and moved to California, I was at a friend's house in London during a giant annual street festival when someone poured a packet of white powder onto a glass table and chopped it into lines. The party guests took turns inhaling them. The young woman beckoned me to the table. I was conscious of standing at a threshold. I had done a lot of drugs by then, but the optics of powder substances retained a distinct illicit frisson and sense of peril. I remembered public health ads on television depicting zombie-like figures who'd ruined their lives through heroin addiction. The drug on the table was cocaine, not heroin, but legally and perceptually they were members of the same taboo class. I took the rolled-up banknote lying on the table and snorted one of the lines. Within seconds a feeling of warmth and calm stillness radiated through me. I noticed how the others were talking faster, compelled to put their racing thoughts into language. I remember listening to a young man deliver what amounted to a sort of personal manifesto, describing his passion for documentary cinema, circling back on how he was uniquely suited for a life committed to that industry. I remember responding only with the nod of my head and the words *yes* and *uh-huh* and my willingness to meet his gaze and listen to him without interruption, yet sensing the great value he was apparently deriving from my stance of rudimentary validation, and observing internally the liberation I felt from any desire to speak, the way the young man's need to be heard formed the mirror image of my silent contentment in attending to him, and noticing myself witness this act of witnessing, in a sort of fractal iteration of consciousness. Everyone did another line of coke. I followed the others through the crowded street to a stage from which tall loudspeakers played house and techno. "This is Sancho Panza," someone said. Time vanished as the music's merger with our dancing bodies formed an imaginary island, a structure perhaps manifesting the mythical *insula* promised to Sancho Panza for his years of service by his insane master, Don Quixote. High on cocaine in a San Francisco bathroom several years later, I remembered that first coke rush in London and an intensity of euphoria that no subsequent usage of that substance could ever quite replicate. The high lasted ten minutes or so and then began to fade. I found the young man with the hoodie and the drugs in his pocket and asked him for more.

About a week later I walked from my apartment to a downtown street corner with a reputation as a hub in the city's drug trade. I was aware of an embarrassing lack of whatever combination of secret winks and street smarts that equipped a person to purchase illegal substances in public from strangers. It was a problem I'd been aware of since college—some stiffness or formality in my bearing that made dealers think I was more likely an undercover cop than a customer. I had no luck at 16th and Mission Streets. I wandered one block to Valencia Street. Two young men in hoodies walked by. One of them muttered something fast under his breath like *weed-pills-rock*—a compound word advertising his wares. "Got any coke?" I said. He shook his head. One of the men beckoned me into an alley. "I ain't got coke," he said, "but I got something better—it lasts longer." He exchanged a smirk and a knowing look with his companion. "Yeah, *way* longer," said the other young man. It was crystal methamphetamine. "Okay, sure, why not," I said. The man named his price. I handed over my cash. He grabbed my hand in a gesture mimicking an energetic handshake in which he transferred a little ziplock bag into my palm.

I was aware of meth's reputation as one of the hardest street drugs available, up there with PCP, the stories of users staying awake on *meth runs* that could last an entire week, at the end of which they were out of their minds, until they crashed and slept for days. Almost everyone I knew had done some kind of recreational substance at least once in their life: at minimum marijuana, and in most instances MDMA, coke, or hallucinogens, at least on special occasions. But I'd never met anyone socially who'd done meth. It was in a category all its own. Of the stigma meted out to drug addicts, those addicted to crystal bore the most ruthless opprobrium. Even crack addicts turned up their noses at meth heads. I had come to understand that there was a sound neurological basis for regarding it with the most serious caution. Among the substances you can put in your brain, methamphetamine is perhaps the most neurotoxic. Brain scans of long-term meth users show parts of the brain with holes in them. I didn't need to read the peer-reviewed neurobiology literature to know that meth would fuck up my brain. Yet that knowledge inspired feelings not of fear or revulsion but of rebellious transgression. *I have crystal.*

It occurred to me that before Miriam and I went back to Burning Man, where I planned to snort my meth, I ought to perform a dress rehearsal with my newfound substance at home. I decided to do a line while I painted the bicycle I intended to bring with me to the desert. I took the baggie out of my pocket. The baggie contained broken shards of a hard, transparent substance. I poured a few shards onto the kitchen table. I crushed the shards into powder. I rolled up a banknote and snorted the powder. I felt a sharp pain at the top of my nose like the stab of a hundred tiny pins. Within seconds I was swaddled by a blanket of euphoria. I went outside and started painting my bicycle. I was conscious of every brushstroke and every detail of the bicycle—the curve of the derailleur, the cylindrical form of the crossbar, the triangles formed by each pair of spokes—as objects that expanded to occupy the entire sphere of my consciousness with a laser-beam-like focus and a feeling of unwavering absorption. On cocaine this state would last for about ten minutes before it faded. On meth it remained constant for several hours.

We drove to the desert. Sometime after the Man burned, I crawled into my tent. I poured out the rest of the meth on a paperback book and snorted it. A sphere of crystalline awareness formed around me. I danced for several hours until the feeling began to fade. I encountered an acquaintance who gave me some Dilaudid, an opioid several times stronger than heroin, which he'd found in the medicine cabinet of an elderly relative lately dead from cancer. Another friend gave me a bump of coke and a swig of water in which he had dissolved some MDMA. I was very high. I heard a rumor that the superstar DJ Armin van Buuren was playing a live set at about four in the morning somewhere on the other side of the desert. I biked through the desert and found a crowd of people dancing. The sun came up. I returned to our camp.

With the sun in my face and drugs in my body, I felt enveloped by warmth and goodness. I understood that my drug taking put me outside the margins of behavior considered acceptable in normal society, and I was aware of the dangers of pushing the limits of what my body could handle. *So what?* I thought. I felt good. I hadn't felt this kind of warmth and goodness in years; perhaps I'd never felt it. I was joyous and jumping and alive. I understood that my feeling derived from the chemicals I had eaten. But everything was chemical—wasn't that the mantra of psychiatry? Sure, meth and Dilaudid carried graver risks than Effexor or Seroquel, but those drugs had done almost nothing good for me, or so I thought, and sometimes seemed to make me feel even worse. *If I'm taking drugs, I may as well do the ones that make me feel good.* In reality, my prescribed psychiatric medication had done something for me—the feeling of the return of an inner brightness I'd experienced on Effexor and Abilify. But it was a mild improvement. My malaise was undiminished. Leaping up and down to techno at sunrise, high on drugs, it was a fake happiness. But fake happiness was surely so much better than real misery. I could feel good—better than good. Transcendent, joyous, free. It was possible for my brain and body to produce these wonderful feelings: *What a discovery!* And wasn't this the point of being alive? What other reason could there be? Surely nobody born on Earth was destined just to struggle through an existence of constant agony, taking pills to numb the pain. I'd stumbled upon the dangerous knowledge understood by every junkie since the beginning of human time. I knew what the lotus-eaters knew. Abandoned by Odysseus on the island with the magic plant that turned his mind into happy mush, the lotus-eater knows his unreal pleasure transports him to much greater wonders than reality could ever match. Odysseus sails off to a home whose existence the lotus-eater has long stopped believing in. *Why set forth on the wine-dark seas and battle monsters when there's this lovely island to stay on?* But the deal the lotus-eater makes by staying on the island is never to return home. To take refuge in the unreal bliss on the island means severing the links to real connection and belonging. It is easy to do so when home seems impossibly distant, perhaps even mythical, a story told by liars to trick a sailor back on board a futile journey of endless cold nights at sea.

Yet the risks were real. I can remember as I finally lay down for a nap around nine in the morning, I could feel my heart beating much too fast. I took some slow deep breaths, but it didn't help. I felt scared. *Oh God, please don't let me die of a heart attack!* I focused again on my breathing, slowing it down, feeling the cycle of my chest moving up and down with each breath, until I felt calmer and then fell asleep.

Nearly everyone went home on Sunday morning after the burning of the Man. Miriam and I stayed to watch the Temple burn. It took place on Sunday evening. The Temple designer modeled his elaborate balsa-wood construction in a form inspired by the temples found in Bali. He offered the Temple to festival participants as a place of mourning. Throughout the week, the wooden surface of the Temple filled with messages in Sharpie or ballpoint pen and handwritten notes and photographs, honoring loved ones now departed from the world. Burners sat on the ground in prayer or meditation, holding each other and sobbing. And then at dusk on Sunday the Temple was set on fire. Burners gathered in a circle a few hundred feet from the inferno. Some called out the names of their beloveds. As I sat beside Miriam, watching the fire, a great wave of grief and shame and sadness overwhelmed me. I wept.

"I'm so ashamed," I said.

"Why, darling?"

"I tried to kill myself."

"But you were depressed," she said. "That was depression."

Miriam held me in her arms. I felt her forgiveness soak through me. I felt the heat from the fire. I heard the sobs of so many others in mourning all around me.

AT WORK, I COULD sense my manager's patience wearing thin. I continued to struggle with the simple tasks she assigned me. I wasn't sure what else to do for work. I searched for other jobs online. In my emails I wore the mask of the Oxford scholar I once had been. I knew—or thought I knew—the effect this mask had on others. But what choice did I really have? Take off the mask? Then what, and who would other people see? Who would I see? It was possible the others knew I was wearing a mask. Maybe they could see the worry lines on my forehead where the mask fit uneasily on my face. *Dear sir or madam, blah blah blah.* I must have applied to fifteen random job listings every day, describing the person I imagined the mask was meant to look like. *I can be like this, or I can be like that,* I said in the mask voice, this character I performed who could take on almost any role. I knew words. Sometimes after a flurry of these emails it was hard to remember whether I wanted any one job more than another. Hard to remember what I wanted other than to be wanted by others. It was pitiful, I thought, how much I depended on this minimal recognition that I mattered and existed. And yet like the bad speed that no one wants to touch until the very end of the night when all the good drugs are gone, I knew this shallow recognition was what I needed to keep my fragile sense of self from crumbling into the familiar feeling of nothingness. Thoughts of alternate future selves flashed from the recesses of my imagination with the desperate ingenuity of C-list Hollywood showrunners crafting lurid plotlines for terminal-phase sitcoms on the eve of network cancellation. Lawyer, doctor, nurse. It occurred to me that I could become an international diplomat. I attended a conference on that field at which the representatives from various prestigious universities stood behind tables stacked with brochures on graduate-degree programs in international relations. *I will be Our Man in North America.* I cycled almost every day between new ideas of what I was supposed to do when I grew up, and when my mind was especially frantic, sometimes more than once per hour. It was exhausting, this performance. When I faced rejection, I felt empty and sad. When I made progress with any of these random schemes, I felt even sadder and emptier, because my success had derived from a phony imitation of a person I had merely assented to performing. It was hard to be sure which sadness was worse. So at night I sat in my room with Charlie. My mind ran in a billion directions, vanishing into imaginary worlds. But in the morning, when Charlie left and I blinked in the sunrise, I felt much, much worse than before.

IN THE FOLLOWING MONTHS my cocaine use ramped up at a rate that ought to have been frightening, had my capacity for fear not been eclipsed by my desire and then need to get high. I started out with gram bags. I proceeded to triple that amount, three-gram bags, or an eighth of an ounce, known in drug lingo as an eight-ball. I met my dealer every week, then twice per week, and then he grew tired of my calls and said I should meet *his* dealer. That was Martha.

"You're not with the FBI or something?" she said.

"No," I said. "Just a customer."

"You don't look like a regular customer."

I mollified her. We went to her apartment. She weighed the cocaine using an electronic scale. I once saw a man there in a dark suit whom I presumed was my dealer's dealer's dealer, an individual who perhaps occupied quite a senior role in the drug-distribution chain, alerting me to the reality that I was crossing a border into territory where the stakes were compounded and unpredictable, possibly launching me into encounters with people who might want to rob me or kill me or send me to prison for a very long time. Once when she handed me an eight-ball, Martha said, "Now, you're not going crazy, are you?" "No," I said. I was. It was my fifth or sixth eight-ball in about a month. *This can't be good for my brain*, I thought. *But . . . but . . . but . . .*

There was always a *but*, a *yet*, an out. I made little deals with myself. *I'll use tonight, then I'll take a day off.* I broke those deals, and made new ones, which I also broke. I was aware of losing control, of neurochemical forces much stronger than my diminished capacity for long-term foresight, or any sense of responsibility to others, driving my actions. I would hit REDIAL to Martha. "I'd like two hundred, please." Then I'd drive to Castro Street, walk upstairs to her apartment, hand over two hundred dollars, go back to my car, make a cursory check that nobody was watching, pour some of the coke on the dash, and snort a line without so much as bothering to chop the rocks into powder.

I would stay awake on coke until 4 a.m., stopping only when the successive diminutions of each euphoric spike flatlined in a stupor. By then all the sharpness and magic from the first few lines of the night had gone, the unmistakable sign that the internal fireworks show was over—the word we used to have in the rave era in England in the '90s was *monged*, a kind of depleted zombie sensation of still being conscious and awake and intoxicated but no longer in the least euphoric or energized; of knowing there was nothing left to be done but sleep and allow at least the minimal degree of neural regeneration necessary to do drugs all over again. Then I would go to bed. I knew that my brain was crying out for rest. But snort cocaine for hours and sleep becomes elusive. I would hunt in the medicine cabinet for Vicodin from an old medical or dental procedure, to try to take the edge off, and then I would lie still until the opioid took effect, my heart thumping, a sense of panic building, sometimes wishing I could wake Miriam up and tell her that I thought I might be having a heart attack, but knowing to do so would entail fessing up to the inexcusable reason, so I just lay there frightened, taking deep breaths, until my pulse slowed down. I was fortunate to have avoided a heart attack, stroke, or seizure. I could have died. I attribute my narrow escape to a combination of relative youth and solid cardiac health, and an element of sheer dumb luck.

I narrowly escaped several other potentially ruinous outcomes. One time I was driving through the city, high, when I accidentally ran a stop sign. A cop pulled me over. I don't remember having drugs in the car, but I'd been up most of the previous night doing coke, and if he'd ordered a drug test, that would have been obvious. I must have looked at least slightly the worse for wear, especially in the eyes of someone like a San Francisco police officer, who sees drunk and high people on the street every day and night and can read the signs of intoxication. "I apologize for running the stop sign, Officer. It was a mistake. I promise I'll never do it again," I said, conscious of enunciating every word in impeccable

BBC English, as if he'd pulled over David Attenborough on a bad day. A posh voice and white skin kept me out of prison.

I also remember making little agreements with myself, at first. *I'll jog round the neighborhood, then I'll treat myself.* I would run at a lumbering, sweaty pace for about twenty minutes nonstop on a short loop that started on the sidewalk outside my apartment. I would head down the street, turn right past the local taqueria, turn right again at the corner store, and then head to a nearby park, before circling back to my apartment. I had gained forty pounds from the combined effects of antipsychotic medication and gluttony. For most of the run, I felt slow, fat, and uncomfortable. But I was moving forward. I was running. My body remembered what to do.

A WHITE SHIMMER APPEARED in the darkness on the screen. Miriam was lying down, her belly covered with translucent gel over which the doctor moved a plastic wand. Our baby would be visible using a new technology known as 4D real-time, which would depict its body in motion, the doctor said. I held Miriam's hand. I looked at the screen above us and gazed at the white shimmer. A pale wash of fuzzy pixels coalesced in human form at 1:54 p.m. I saw a face. I saw a nose. I saw a tiny arm, moving through the void to the right side of the face, like a wave. *Hello, Mama. Hello, Dada.* Seven ounces, the doctor said. Heart rate normal, the doctor said: 135 beats per minute. A girl. Miriam cried happy tears. We kissed. I shook the doctor's hand. I felt a new emotion. It had the echo of feelings long dormant, a sense of wonder at the mystery of creation, the way I'd felt as a boy, staring into the night sky, imagining distant worlds, but mixed with a feeling that seemed altogether novel, the awareness of joining together in the mystery, of participating now as Being's coauthor, as if what had emerged in the darkness from the shimmer was my own embryonic consciousness becoming real in time.

Late at night I would sit by my computer, pouring white crumbs of cocaine onto my desk and chopping them into short, skinny columns.

How I yearned to recapture the rapture of the first one! It had the excitement of Christmas morning, the wonder of a euphoric and radiant present, wrapped around me. *Everything is connected*, I would think, rushing down some manic path of introspective derangement in which my every random thought felt interlinked and revelatory.

I spent many such late nights writing a short story about a time traveler. The action shifted between ancient Egypt and contemporary London. It involved the time traveler's quest to recover a famous lost manuscript, destroyed in the burning ruins of the Library of Alexandria. By two in the morning I found it hard to focus. The logical paradoxes entailed in time travel proved impossible to resolve. The drugs made my head hurt. But there was an easy remedy to feeling bad on drugs: more drugs. *Don't worry about what this must be doing to your brain. Don't vex about tomorrow morning. Do another line.*

The self is also a kind of line, a trail linking the feeling of a unitary conscious being across space and time. For the bundle of thought and feeling that you experienced as *you* five years ago and now, for the self at home and at work and walking among strangers in the street, convention identifies a single legal person, the entity denoted in the English language by a short skinny column: *I*.

Once upon a time, every one of us was two. I was Mummy-and-me, hyphenate twin souls linked by connections first umbilical and then emotional. Late at night with Charlie I felt something like that unity again, or how I wished it might have been. Chop, chop, chop: snort another line, and the path I followed traveled back through time, reminding me of how it felt to be vital, joyous, connected. But follow the line that leads into a delusory heaven and you cut the links that keep your feet upon the ground. The me-with-Charlie and me-with-Miriam split into two separate people. I chopped up myself. I chopped up the truth. I chopped up my dignity.

I stopped trusting myself. Perhaps I never had. I had minimal confidence that if I planned to do something, that intention was something I could count on sustaining even hours into the future. If I made any sort of plan, in my own mind my words had terms and conditions attached to them, inscribed outside the realm of discourse in six-point font, absolving me from the responsibility to follow through on what I said as a result of conditions including, but not limited to: drug relapse or overdose; feeling hungover and grouchy; feelings of depressive implosion, boredom, procrastination, distraction, spacing out; willful disavowal of my commitment due to resentment projected upon others from ancient unhealed emotional injuries; quitting my job and fleeing for the hills; psychiatric confinement; incarceration; self-injury; or death by suicide. Those were the terms I lived by, despite my awareness that they were unknown to other people, who would never have consented to such terms had they known about them. I didn't like myself for living this way; at times I disliked my disliking. Sometimes I had memories of a little Catholic altar boy in England, the boy with his hand up with the right answer, the boy racing across the field to the eighty-yard finish line on Sports Day, and I was aware of the man I had become, and how far I had stumbled from any path into a future self that the boyhood me would have considered noble or honorable or worthy, and my heart fell to the ground and would not lift up again.

I knew that Charlie and I could never last. But so long as my secret romance lasted, I resolved to make the most of it. Everyone was so relieved to hear that I was feeling good again. I saw no reason to disappoint them. Miriam asked me why there was blood on my pillow. "Allergies," I said. Another time she found a rolled-up banknote with crumbs of cocaine inside it on my desk. "Left over from Burning Man," I said.

"I was five months pregnant—we were getting ready to start a family, or I thought we were," she told me years later. "Absolutely the last thing I could have imagined was that you were doing drugs. You were in your office half the night, writing, and you seemed so into it, and I was so relieved you weren't depressed anymore—that's what I wanted to believe, what I had to believe. The signs you were an addict were staring me in the face. But I couldn't make the connections, because it would have meant really knowing something I didn't want to know." I didn't want to know either.

On some level I must have understood that doing drugs all night at best guaranteed jeopardizing my marriage and at worst risked overdose and death. I dwelt in a kind of twilight between knowing and not knowing. We both did. Yet it soon became impossible for either of us to run away from the reality of my addiction. At about seven on a weekday morning in early December 2005 I was hunched over a fat line of white powder on my desk. Miriam walked through the door, a dressing gown over her big pregnant belly. "Oh my God," she said, seeing the drugs on the desk. "You have to be fucking kidding me."

I had done nothing whatsoever to conceal what I was doing. I hadn't even bothered to close the door. On an unconscious level, perhaps, I had wanted her to find me. Needed her to find me and put a stop to the insanity. She grabbed the baggie and emptied its contents into the toilet. "What are you doing?" I said. I couldn't believe she'd wasted a whole bag of perfectly decent drugs.

I drove to work. Within the hour, my brain—deprived of the daily high dose of cocaine that over the past few months had altered the way my mood and motivation were regulated by the neurotransmitter dopamine—entered a withdrawal state that has a psychological quality comparable to but in excess of extreme thirst or hunger. The conventional word for this state is *craving*. The word doesn't do justice to the level of torment entailed. My consciousness collapsed into an awareness of not being high and an urge to reverse that situation immediately, a distress compounded by the knowledge that my secret was now out, and for the first time I was facing—in Miriam's threat of divorce—what appeared to be real consequences for my addiction, an outcome that was unbearable to me. My mind ran back and forth between the picture of a life without Miriam, high, and a picture of life with her, sober but craving drugs.

Images of doing coke flashed into my mind's eye like a virtual-reality simulation. I could see the whole scene in front of me, almost as if it was actually happening: the line chopped up on the table, the incomparable combination of immense relief and satisfaction as the drug absorbed through my nasal membranes and the shiny inner lights came back on. All I needed to do was hit REDIAL to reach Martha. The images circled in my mind.

Hello, said Charlie. *I'm here. You know you can call me any time, right?*

Yes, Charlie. But you'll fuck up my life.

Hmmm . . . Let's not get carried away worrying about that right now, okay? Focus on the packet. Open it up. Done that? Good. You know what comes next. Tap those little babies on the desk and chop, chop, chop. Now. BREATHE! Ah . . . Here it comes . . . just—so—good. Isn't that worth it? Don't you remember me?

Yes, Charlie.

Aren't you—hitting—redial—to Martha—right—this—instant?

BY THE TIME I flew my mother over from England about a month later for Christmas I had relapsed and was using cocaine again. I drove to the airport. I stood waiting in the arrivals lobby until she came shuffling through the door with a large leather briefcase in her hand. She looked much smaller than I remembered. It was beyond all understanding, how the lovely lady who sang the ballads I remembered from long ago had turned into this old woman, talking gibberish. In the morning I drove her fifty miles south to see the elephant seals that live on the beach there. I had run out of drugs and couldn't get back to the city fast enough. I left her with Miriam and went to see Martha and bought an eight-ball. By the time Mum and I entered the lobby of the De Young Museum in Golden Gate Park I was already good and high. When I felt myself descending from the peak of euphoria, I excused myself to visit the bathroom. I poured a fat line on the white ceramic surface of the toilet and snorted the drugs into my body. As I left the bathroom and went back to the exhibits, my gaze was drawn upward by a gigantic Gerhard Richter canvas that covered an entire wall, depicting the atomic structure of strontium titanate. *Everything is made of protons and electrons . . . strontium . . . me . . . Mum . . .*

Before leaving, we visited the gift shop. I found a book about Australian Aboriginal art. It contained pictures of lizards and birds and kangaroos, drawn from multicolored dots. According to Aboriginal cosmology, all reality emerged from the Dreaming, the book's introduction stated. Dots . . . protons . . . I felt my heart racing. "We should go," I said and led my mother to the car. We were somewhere near Market Street when a pressure began building in the side of my head. *Oh Jesus, I'm having a stroke—a seizure—a heart attack.* I pulled the car to the side of the road. I got out of the car and sat down on the street. I felt my heart beat faster. I was breathing fast but felt like I was suffocating. The street and everything in it faded into an unreal distance. *I'm going to die here—how fucking stupid.* "Are you okay?" said a stranger, catching sight of me sitting on the ground. "Do you need an ambulance?" "No," I said. "What's wrong with you?" my mother said. "Nothing," I said. My heart rate slowed, and my panic subsided with it. I got back into the car and drove us back to my apartment in the Mission.

Charlie, you're a liar. How can you say you love someone and treat them like that? I'd taken drugs because I wanted to feel joyous and alive and free. But in the car that night, verging on cocaine overdose, I felt trapped and frightened.

Goodbye, Charlie.

I HEARD A CRY and saw her pink face and half-inch of light brown hair and large feet and the engorgement of her lips. I put out my finger, and she clasped it with her tiny hand. I can remember my awareness of the magnitude of what was occurring, of life restructuring around a division between the world before the birth of our daughter and the new world whose threshold we had now passed beyond. We stayed in the hospital for a week while Miriam recovered from her C-section. When we left with our daughter in the car seat, as I gripped the steering wheel, it struck me as remarkable that a person didn't need special qualifications for this sort of thing, meaning fatherhood—how strange it was that I needed a license to drive but not to bear the primary responsibility for a newborn human life.

In the first days and weeks of my daughter's life the cosmos shrunk to the cradle: the world beyond the nursery fell away. It was as if the feeling of being with our daughter had pulled me into a kind of dream, a space between baby and parent where the two of us ran together.

On a rare sober night that summer, I was holding my daughter in my arms when I felt an astonishing new emotion. The feeling started in my heart, a tender warmth that then radiated all through me and then between the two of us and then seemed to pervade the room, merging with the pinkish-purple luminosity from my daughter's night-light. The entire universe seemed to fall away, leaving the two of us there, my daughter and me, in the nursery. I felt as if I had been running, lost in a dark forest of the mind, when a path appeared with a sign that said THIS WAY. I looked into her eyes. *I love you. I will protect you.*

I had long assumed that drugs and alcohol helped me feel something. But in truth, they had the opposite effect. A fake chemical connection is a poor substitute for a real and living one. A drug high is indeed a kind of feeling, but it tends to screen more subtle emotions from awareness.

I decided to quit drugs. I thought that I could keep on drinking.

··

I lay back in the passenger seat. An atmosphere of menace pervaded the car interior. It was around ten at night. I felt nauseated from the wine I had been drinking nonstop since we arrived five hours earlier at a friend's party celebrating Yom Kippur, the Jewish day of atonement. I was almost too drunk to speak, a sorry candidate for any sort of reconciliation. Booze was a poor substitute for Charlie. My first few slurps would give me a bit of a buzz, but as I kept on boozing, the buzz would fade away, and the lights turn off inside me, rendering me dizzy and half-asleep. As the car crossed over the Golden Gate Bridge and swung hard onto Lombard Street, I realized that I was about to vomit.

"Pull over," I said. Miriam stopped the car. I opened the door and fell to the ground on my hands and knees. The contents of my stomach erupted in spasms upon the ground. I got back into the car, and Miriam drove us home. Her face registered not anger but disgust. "I'm done," she said. "This time I'm really done."

I understand. I don't want her to leave. But I do understand. Who could blame her? She's coped with me suicidal. Then as a cokehead. Can I really now expect her to put up with me as a garden-variety drunk, puking up my guts on the street?

Soon, it appeared, I would truly be alone. Lost. Abandoned. A failure. Even if Miriam could tolerate such a broken man as her husband, our darling daughter surely deserved a sober and responsible dad. "I'll get help. I promise," I said. "I don't believe you," she said. I wasn't sure I believed myself.

FROM THE CITY, I followed the coastal highway south. I kept my eyes on the road and my mind on anything but me. Thoughts spun around my frightened consciousness. *What a fool I am. What an idiot. I did this to myself.* I found a motel with an available room. I carried my bag inside the room. I lay down and fell asleep. I woke in the early morning. I drove to the forest. I parked in a campground. I could see the other runners standing near the trailhead in the dawn sunlight. I picked up a little piece of paper with a number on it. I attached the paper to my shorts with safety pins. I went and stood with the runners. I listened to an older man with tan skin and calves like cantaloupes talking to the people standing next to him. He was running the marathon, he said. It was good training for a fifty-miler. One of the very fit people said his wife had once run a hundred miles. He meant nonstop. He had run with her from mile 75 to the end. It was madness to behold, he said. She was a warrior. She ran all day until the sun went down and then she kept on running. Sometime in the dark night he watched her stumble and catch herself from falling to the ground. "I fell asleep," she told him.

"That's what my wife does for fun," he said. "You wouldn't know it to look at her, but she's this insane badass who can run in the mountains for thirty hours straight."

There were others like her, the man said. The ultrarunners. They were crazy people. Crazy in a good way. They took their crazy and put it to use. They ran until they were on their knees and puking up their guts and crying and then they got up and kept on running.

"Incredible," I said. I could picture the warrior woman of whom the man spoke. I didn't believe in much of anything, back then. But if I had met this ultrarunner woman, I would have wanted to shake her by the hand and say, *Ma'am, I salute you. In a world of broken promises and bullshit, you have done something real. A hundred fucking miles. There could be some global decree from the pope and the president saying you were a no-good piece of shit and what those schmucks said wouldn't matter in the slightest.* "I ran a hundred miles, dude—what did YOU do?"

In the silence of the forest nobody knew my name. I was the number pinned on my shorts. I was the sweat on my face. I was the feeling of my chest moving and the sound of every inhale and exhale. I was the breeze and the sun and the birdsong. All that mattered was forward motion.

How could you do that to someone you love?

Left, right, left, right. Silence.

Huff-puff, thump-thump, huff-puff, thump-thump.

A breeze, a whisper.

I'm done with you. An echo. A sigh. The crunch of feet on gravel.

Hello, says the bird, *hello. Listen,* say the trees. *We are many. We were here long before all the sad old voices that call you back to the ruins.*

Coo-coo, says the bird. *Hush now. This way—look.* A path appears. *I am before you and beside you and below you and within you.*

IX

Neptune

Namu Kie Butsu

From the summit it's about a thousand-foot descent to the next aid station. My light-headedness fades as Emily and I lose altitude. At the aid station, I sit down in one of the camping chairs beneath the blazing sun. There are five or six others sitting in chairs with dazed looks on their faces. A bearded fellow carves a hole in an apple with a knife, fills the hole with marijuana, and lights it. I can't imagine wanting to get high here. I'm already high. LSD was never quite this good. Take acid, and you drop through a rabbit hole into Wonderland. Or hell. This state of mind feels a bit like Wonderland too. But it's different. What do you call the place where the sun feels really hot and the creek feels really cold and food tastes really good and your loved ones feel so precious you want to weep with joy? Reality.

Later, ahead of us on the trail, I can see a man plodding uphill with the slow cadence of a Zen monk performing walking meditation. I exchange a fist bump with this mountain Buddha. His face is red with sunburn and the crumpled look of a person who hasn't slept in several days. His features form into a half-smile, conveying a hardship borne with serenity. His brow then furrows with the intimation of a mind turned quizzical, inspired, perhaps, by the emergence of other human minds in proximity to him, the opportunity afforded by the chance to break his silence, pulling him from the long reverie in which he had been hitherto suspended, for hours if not for days, perhaps his entire life.

"Was there sunscreen at that aid station?" says Mountain Buddha. "Yes," I say. "Back there?" he says, pointing down the hill—the aid station was miles away. "Yes," I say. "So you mean," he says, "that if I need sunscreen, I need to go back down there?" "Yes," I say. Mountain

Buddha nods, as if in recognition of a noble truth, already known to the Buddhas of the past. Mountain Buddha then turns to face the steep trail ahead of us. He points his finger at the forest. "When we get to the top of this hill," he says, "do you happen to remember, might there be a parking lot?" "I don't know," I say. "I haven't been there yet." I doubt the existence of mountain parking lots. Mountain Buddha nods. He has understood something. Mountain Buddha smiles. "Right," he says. "Because if there really was a parking lot—that would be déjà vu." I say goodbye to Mountain Buddha and hike onward through the trees.

IT'S THE MIDDLE OF the afternoon, and I'm shuffling on an exposed section of trail underneath the baking High Sierra sun. I can't remember that I've ever felt quite so utterly exhausted. It's hard to think straight. Emily and I stop at a creek to refill our water bottles. There are another couple of runners sitting down by the water. I recognize one of them. It's Don from Belize. "How's it going, man?" I say. "Hot," he says. "Tired." "Me too," I say. There's a certain comfort in solidarity. He looks how I feel: sleepy-eyed, frazzled, and drained. You reach a point in this sort of state when it stops making sense to keep struggling forward, getting slower and weaker by the step. This kind of fatigue has a nonnegotiable quality. There is the kind of tired you can power through. Eat some food and douse your head in creek water and off you go again. But there is another kind of tired for which the only remedy is sleep. Like a car with an overheated engine, you need to park your brain in the breakdown lane for a while so the circuits can cool off. *I need to lie down. Right now.* "Nap time," I tell Emily. "Okay," she says. I lie down on the ground by the side of the trail, underneath a tree. Staring up at the leaves and the little patches of blue sky between them, I don't have a care in the world. A feeling of lovely contentment and peace washes through me. Sometimes I think the point of all my running is to remember what it feels like to stop and rest. I mean *really* rest. Everything settles and slows . . . down. There's nothing I need to do. Nowhere else I need to be. If I imagine a perfect death, it would be like this, looking up at the leaves and sky, and feeling this delicious sense of absolute completion. I close my eyes.

A MAN SITS DOWN beneath a tree. He closes his eyes in meditation. *I will not leave here until I understand the nature of my mind*, he thinks. He follows his thoughts for hours as they run through his mind. His mind settles. The morning comes. He understands the nature of suffering and liberation. All phenomena are subject to decay. Everything arises and falls away: kings and the great towers of the wealthy and every instant of time. Run after the moment just gone and you might as well chase a ghost. The man stands up. He shares his understanding with others. They call him the awakened one, the Buddha. They learn how to still their minds in *dhyana*, concentration. His followers travel north from India to China and from China to Japan. In China *dhyana* becomes *chan*, and in Japan *chan* becomes *zen*. In the 1960s a Zen priest called Shunryu Suzuki flew from Japan to San Francisco, to found the first Zen temple in the Western Hemisphere, San Francisco Zen Center. Shunryu Suzuki taught Gyugaku Hoitsu. Gyugaku Hoitsu taught Hakuryu Sojun. Hakuryu Sojun taught Shosan Gigen. Shosan Gigen taught me.

I first went to the Zen Center when I was a couple of weeks sober, to a meditation meeting for people in recovery from addiction. I entered a hall with round cushions on the floor. People were sitting on the cushions with their legs crossed in front of them. The room was very quiet. No one said a word. At the front of the room there was an older man with a dark blue piece of cloth hung around his neck. Behind him was a line of tall Buddha statues. "Find a comfortable way to sit still," he said. "I can see some of you are sitting in half-lotus like me. That's fine. But if you can't sit in lotus position, it's no big deal. That's not the point. The point is to sit. Then just pay attention to your breath. When you breathe in, notice that. When you breathe out, notice that. It might help to count your exhalations from one to five. If you lose count, don't worry—just go back to one. If you reach five, go back to one. For most of us, what you'll then notice is your mind, running about all over the place. The traditional Zen picture for this is a wild ox. We try to train the ox by putting boundaries around it. The boundary in zazen is your attention. The mind runs somewhere else—come back to this breath right now. And that's really all there is to it."

Someone dimmed the lights. I heard a bell ring. The room was quiet. I observed my breath. The ox of my mind crashed through the barrier of my attention. I nodded off. Minutes felt like hours. My knees hurt. The pattern on the carpet looked like it was breathing.

It was raining hard when I woke some months later on the morning of the daylong retreat. My clothes were damp when I entered the zendo and sat down on one of the cushions. I survived the first forty-minute period of zazen, shivering. After that there was a five-minute period of *kinhin*, walking meditation. It was a relief to stand and move my legs even in this weird slow walk the *kinhin* involved. I struggled through a second and third period of zazen.

By the end of the third period daylight was streaming through the windows in the zendo. I could tell it was a sunny day outside. I thought of Miriam and our daughter at home. *Come back to the breath*—isn't that what I'm supposed to do? The longer I counted my breath, the more I thought of Miriam and our beautiful little girl. In the early afternoon the retreat organizers made an announcement. You could speak to a priest about how the retreat was going for you, in a formal meeting called *dokusan*. "Sign me up," I said. The priest they sent me to was Shosan Gigen.

"I'm thinking about my wife and baby daughter," I said. "I know I'm not supposed to. But I am."

"Perhaps that is your practice now," she said. "To be with them. Not here in the temple. The zendo isn't going anywhere. But your daughter will only be two for a little while. Go to them."

I left the temple and ran the two miles home.

A decade later I went back. I had been studying Zen for several years by then. I could sit still and meditate all day. I had studied the Bodhisattva Precepts, the ethical principles of Zen Buddhism: *Don't kill. Don't lie. Don't steal. Don't gossip. Don't intoxicate your mind with substances.* I wanted to make a formal commitment as a Zen Buddhist to live by those vows. In Zen this involves a ceremony called *jukai*, in which you make the following pledge: "All of my ancient twisted karma, from beginningless greed, hate, and delusion, born through body, speech, and mind, I now fully avow." You accept who you are. You look back at the path that got you here, back to your birth, and your ancestors, back through time, all the steps that led up to you. You acknowledge them and walk forward with dignity.

Early in my study of Zen I came across the idea of the Four Dignities. It conveys the idea that every moment of your life presents an opportunity for the kind of open, focused awareness cultivated in meditation. The Four Dignities are the four basic postures of the body: sitting, standing, walking, lying down. Later it occurred to me that there are an infinite number of dignities. There is the dignity of laundry. The dignity of brushing your teeth. The dignity of being human. I like to think of running as the Fifth Dignity.

To prepare for *jukai*, Shosan told me, I would need to sew a *rakusu*, a rectangular piece of cloth that hangs around the neck, like the one I had seen the teacher wearing the first time I went to the Zen Center.

I went to the Zen temple sewing class and started stitching. It was the first time I'd sewn anything since I made a penguin in Mrs. Mahon's class when I was nine. Like almost everything else from Cannon Road, the penguin had disappeared. Sometimes in between my stiches I would picture my lost penguin and the boy I once was who had lost him. "While you are sewing," said Shosan, "repeat this mantra in your mind: *Namu kie Butsu. Namu kie Ho. Namu kie So.*"

It was Japanese that referred to the Three Refuges of Buddha, Dharma, and Sangha. *Butsu* is Buddha, the possibility of liberation. *Ho* is Dharma, the teachings about that possibility. *So* is Sangha, the community of people who aspire to live by those teachings. *Namu kie*

Butsu: I take refuge in the Buddha. *Namu kie Ho*: I take refuge in the Dharma. *Namu kie So*: I take refuge in the Sangha.

I told Shosan about my plan to run around Lake Tahoe.

"Take refuge when you're running," she said. "Take refuge in the mountain."

..

The forest feels infinite. I hike through the trees, contemplating the possibility that I will never leave them. Everything hurts. My feet, my legs, my back, my shoulders, my neck, my lips, my tongue. I'm around 130 miles in. It's hard enough to contemplate the thousands of steps I'll need to make it to the next aid station, 5 miles from here, let alone the 70 miles still left after that. *Namu . . . kie . . . Butsu.* Here I am, in the forest. Yes, there is pain. But beauty too. *Don't run away from it. Turn toward it. Don't block it out. Don't wish anything were otherwise. There's nothing else but this—step—now. Namu . . . kie . . . Butsu.* I turn toward my shin pain. I turn toward my blistered feet and ulcerated tongue and sunburn and my stale-sweat stink and the trees and dirt and sky and the pain again and the sky again and this step and now and pain and beauty and Earth and heaven and the left foot and the right one. There is nothing outside this—step—now. I have always been here. I will always be here. Every step is home.

Home Again

I drove to the ocean. It was still dark in the early morning. Sometimes the water was invisible beneath a shroud of fog. Other times the sky was clear. I could see the stars and moon. I understood that the stars had always been there. But I had never seen them shining with such brightness. Sometimes I would watch the giant cargo ships on the dark horizon, arriving at the Golden Gate after their long journey across the ocean from Asia, illuminated like Christmas trees in pink and purple lights. I felt my feet squish on the soft, wet sand and listened to the roar of the wind and felt on my face the cold, damp air that smelled of kelp and burnt firewood. Pelicans flew in a triangular formation low above the water. I saw satellites drifting in the blackness high above me. In the rooms of Alcoholics Anonymous I had heard about the need to find a power greater than myself. I came to believe in what I could see and feel and touch and smell and hear. I believed in the smell of seaweed and the cry of seagulls and the twinkle of Orion. Sometimes memories of the distant past bubbled into awareness as the rhythm of my feet on the ground reminded me of rhythms and feelings long forgotten and presumed irrecoverable. *Home again, home again, jiggety-jig*, I thought. It was what we had said when we got home. I would hear the crunch of our green Citroën on the gravel driveway in Cannon Road and all of us would say it together: me and Mummy and Daddy and Sebastian. We were home again. I was home again.

At the start, running felt effortful and awkward, reminiscent of what I'd experienced when I was learning to drive as a teenager: a discombobulated sequence of movements I consciously willed into being one at a time, until the movements eventually burned grooves into my cerebellum and became as automatic as breathing. But over time running became effortless. I found an easy pace, and I didn't feel out of breath.

It felt as natural as walking, and I noticed how it helped me to stand tall when I ran, shoulders relaxed, arms held loose, noticed the way my jaw clenched if I started obsessing about something, and how to relax my jaw was to unclench my mind. I learned how to take care of a sore calf and an inflamed and tender mid-foot, to understand what this pain was asking of me, and how to listen to it like the cry of a frightened child. I felt how the daily run put structure in the day, formed a rhythm that other parts of my life started to beat in time with. I learned to run farther and farther through the hills, and I found out how after being outside in the cold fog and going home and getting into the bath, I was wrapped in a warmth that soaked into every cell and every wounded part of me.

As I ran in the dark on the wet sand, I would feel the Earth coming up to meet me with every footfall, a rhythm of sound and motion that held me and rocked me, as if the solid ground became my mother's arms, wrapped around the infant I once had been. "I don't know where I'm headed," I would say, and Earth said: *This way.* "I don't know who I am," I said, and Earth said: *Feel your left foot landing and now your right. That's it. Feel your chest rise and fall. Feel your arms swing back and forth. Listen to the wind. Behold the birds in the air above you. Pay attention to the moon. Observe the gap between takeoff and landing, the space when you are airborne, yet how I come back to you with each step. You can trust that I am with you. I will never go away. I am Earth.*

NEPTUNE WAS THE GOD of the sea. In the ancient world, the sea was the chaotic realm that stood between the known world and distant lands. To seek far-off shores, you had to get on a boat. You also had to cross the sea when you wanted to return home again. Both voyages were risky. You could drown. You could find yourself shipwrecked and alone on a strange island. You could run out of fresh water and start drinking salt water and go insane. But water was also the medium of transformation. The literal and symbolic domain where the soul could seek new lands and find its way back home. Find your way to safe harbor and you can heal. You can start to make sense of the times you felt at sea. Chaotic memories and frantic thinking can settle into a feeling of coherence and centered calm.

That feeling comes from the kind of reorganization in the brain and mind that becomes possible in a restorative environment: someplace where you can run free. Experimental studies of nonhuman animals yield persuasive evidence illuminating some of the key chemical mechanisms involved. Some years ago a group of neurobiologists assembled a group of mouse depressives.[14] When a mouse is hung upside down by its tail, it tries to wriggle away. If the mouse soon abandons its escape attempt, it is understood to be depressed.

The scientists put the sad mice in a playground. They had never dreamed such freedom might be possible! The mice skipped and scampered about. Their depression faded away. The scientists looked inside their brains. They were interested in a chemical called brain-derived neurotrophic factor, or BDNF. It helps new cells grow in a region of the brain called the hippocampus that underpins the capacity to learn and remember. After the mice ran out to play, they had more BDNF in their brains. Further research has shown that running has a similar effect on human brains. When you run, you remember what it feels like to be free.

THERE IS A SONG I used to sing in the choir at Glide Memorial before I went into the hospital that went like this:

> *We fall down, but we get up*
> *For a saint is just a sinner*
> *Who fell down*
> *And got up.*

I was no saint. But I did get up. Nothing had prepared me for the emotions that flooded my awareness when I put down the chemical shield I'd so long held against them. Abstinence from booze and drugs was hard enough. I missed Charlie. Without her arms wrapped around me, I was alone again, naked and afraid. Every day on the inside I battled with the urge to get high, the knowledge of the calamitous consequences of doing so, memories of the degradation to which I'd succumbed. But the real challenge of living sober had less to do with the absence of intoxication and more to do with the presence of feelings I was ill-equipped to handle. Everything felt uncertain. I didn't want to die anymore. I wanted to live, but I didn't know how. I was fat, drug-addicted, lonely, scared, ashamed, and angry.

I knew big words. But nothing I had ever learned from my parents or my teachers or in the thousands of books I'd read had equipped me to handle life. If the School of Life gave classes on how a sad person was supposed to avoid turning into a suicidal drug addict, I had missed them.

I EMBRACED THE LIFE of a distance runner with the repentant zeal of the sinner who fell down and got up again. I read all the running books. I read *Runner's World*, *Running Times*, and *Trail Runner* magazines. I read every running blog on the internet. I watched all the good running movies, then all the bad ones, then random online montages of unedited running footage, cut with cheesy '80s rock anthems that made me weep with a new emotion. It wasn't sadness. It wasn't joy. The closest term I could find to describe the feeling was what the Japanese call *mono no aware*, literally "the pathos of things," a bittersweet awareness of the transience of all phenomena. I was alive and healthy, and I could run all day in the forest and the mountains. It couldn't last. One day I would die. But what a marvel it was in the moment at last to really feel alive!

I ran every day. I ran when I was hot and when I was cold and when I was hungry and thirsty and tired and hurting and delirious. I ran until I didn't want to run anymore and then I kept on running. I ran until all my sweat and sore muscles and the stronger legs and lungs and willpower that came from all those millions of steps on the road and through the hills and woods had given me a kind of knowledge, in the way the body knows things, that feelings were survivable.

It's going to be all right, my body came to understand. *Feel the feeling. Breathe in. Breathe out. Stay with it.* There were names for the sensations that for so long had struck me outside conscious awareness as impulses to get high or leave the country or kill myself.

Hello, sadness. Hello, fear. Hello, shame. I can hear you. Sure, I'll listen to your bad ideas. Sadness, you want me to lie down and never get up again. I'm getting up. Fear, you want me to get the hell out of here. I feel you, man. But I'm staying. Shame, you want me to go hide in the corner and keep my mouth shut. I want to go play outside with the others in the sun. It's dark inside here with you, old buddy. So goodbye. I imagine you'll be back. I confess, my heart is rather full these days. But you're always welcome down in the basement.

Years later I was staying in a house by the Northern Californian coast when a little bird flew in but couldn't find its way out again. I opened a window and a large sliding door, but the bird kept flying against a single spot on a closed window near the ceiling, far out of reach above me, smashing its head against the glass, over and over again. Miriam and my children and I called to the bird. "This way!" we said, pointing to the way out through the open door. But the bird kept flying back and forth, smashing its head against the glass. I found a stepladder and climbed to the area near the ceiling and the bird. I cupped my hands to form a sphere in which I held the frightened bird. It went limp. "It's dead!" I felt so sad for the bird. I hadn't meant to kill it. But after all that thrashing against the window, the shock of my hands had overwhelmed the poor little thing. I took the dead bird outside and laid it on the ground. I sat with Miriam and our children looking at the ocean. "I feel sorry for the bird," my daughter said. "Me too," I said. Time passed—perhaps twenty minutes, as we sat there looking at the ocean and feeling sorry about the bird. Then we saw its lifeless body start to twitch. Then the twitching exploded into a kind of shudder that became a flutter of wings and the bird flapped away and was gone. The bird had been frozen. In the face of overwhelming stress, an ancient evolutionary defense mechanism, deep in the core of its nervous system, had kicked in to paralyze the bird. In the first days and weeks of sobriety, I could feel my nervous system twitching and shuddering as the frozen state of drug and alcohol dependence began to thaw.

From the bible of the sport, a book called *Lore of Running*, by the exercise physiologist Tim Noakes, I gleaned the basic principles of how the body adapts to training. I felt some affinity with Steve Austin, hero of *The Six Million Dollar Man*, a TV show I'd liked watching as a boy, in the opening credits of which we learn he had been an astronaut, nearly killed in a horrible accident, then reassembled by hi-tech boffins into a cybernetically enhanced version of his former self: "Steve Austin, astronaut. A man barely alive. Gentlemen, we can rebuild him. We have the technology. We have the capability to build the world's first bionic man. Steve Austin will be that man. Better than he was before. Better, stronger, faster."

I decided that I would rebuild myself through running. *Jason Thompson, disheveled Englishman. I have the books and blogs and videos. I will become a bionic version of myself. Better. Stronger. Faster.*

I ran a marathon. I ran fifty kilometers. I ran fifty miles, and then a hundred miles. Running restored rhythm to my life. For as long as I could remember, I had never felt like anything in my experience was truly trustworthy. I was always afraid that the ground could collapse at any second and I'd have to run away again. A boy afraid of the Bomb became a man afraid of his own mind. It's impossible to trust other people until you can trust yourself. Running made my own experience trustworthy. Every step was much like the last one, and the feelings in a run followed a reliable sequence, from the sluggish, awkward inertia of the first ten minutes, to the sensation of everything loosening up, to the long stretch of dreaming and flowing, to the creep of fatigue, to the warm afterglow that would last well into the morning. I came to know this rhythm in the intuitive way that you know how to ride a bike or sew or drive a car or dance the salsa: the kind of how-to knowledge that, given enough repetition, gets folded into muscle memory. You learn the steps and practice, practice, practice, and soon enough you don't have to worry that you'll ever forget them. The body remembers, so the thinking mind doesn't need to.

I learned how to relax in the midst of intense sensation, how to notice spots of tension, like a clenched jaw or tightness in my shoulders, and release them. I learned that it was better, feeling pain, to contain it in awareness, with a sense of lightness, not checking out from it, not punishing myself, but just noticing it, relaxing around it, being with it, staying with it. I noticed how after running fast like this all my other runs felt easier and easier. I noticed that the willingness to stay with the experience, to set an intention to do something hard, however arbitrary, and then do it, created a sense of internal trustworthiness, feelings of confidence and competence, a kind of embodied knowing that I could stay with not just running but anything. Anything at all.

After two years of running and staying sober, I felt more solid on the inside than I could remember feeling in a long time. I wasn't depressed. I didn't have any cravings for drugs or alcohol. I had found quieter and more reliable sources of joy: the feeling of flying through the woods and hills; the feeling of togetherness with Miriam and our two-year-old daughter; the deep fulfillment of teaching students in my new job at an elementary school. I trusted that I wasn't going to drink or do drugs again. I trusted that I could pick a point two miles away and run toward it and get there. I trusted that if I told you I'd see you tomorrow, I wasn't going to wake up in the morning depressed or freaking out and need to bail.

But when I remembered the dark ages of my addiction, I felt disgusted and ashamed. Images of my cokehead liar self getting high in my room in the wee hours while Miriam was pregnant would flash into my mind's eye with a rush of revulsion. *What the hell was I doing? What was I even thinking?* It was time I looked back again, to follow the trail from the stable ground I'd found back through the fog of addiction, to the hospital, to all my years of running away.

I had heard Jim speak in meetings for about six months before I asked him to be my sponsor. He had a laid-back and honest quality that I found very appealing. He was born poor and orphaned in his early teens, he told me later. He joined a violent gang. Years passed. He remembered the rage and suffering of his frightened boyhood through an amnesiac screen of booze and drugs and denial. A day of reckoning arrived. He stood at the threshold of either redemption or annihilation. He chose to acknowledge the reality of his past. He did not do so alone. He followed the steps that others had trod before him: his sponsor, his sponsor's sponsor, back through the generations, to the origin of the fellowship.

"I have two questions you need to answer if you want me to sponsor you," said Jim, when we met for the first time in his apartment.

"Go ahead," I said.

"Number one: Are you willing to do *anything* to stay sober?"

"Yes," I said.

"Number two: Are you going to waste my time?"

"No," I said.

How different this interaction with Jim felt compared to my experiences with Dr. Jensen and Dr. Browning. His directness communicated a message I had not absorbed before. It was as if I were sleepwalking, and about to stumble off a balcony, and he shook me awake. Three parts of what he said stood out. *Willing*: it was up to me. Nobody else was going to do it. *Anything*: I had to put my sobriety first. It might be hard. *Waste my time*: He was a person too. This wasn't just about me. It was about us. *I commit to you; you commit to me.*

I was okay with steps one and two, the bit about powerlessness and needing a higher power. But after that, the twelve steps got gnarly. There was the suggestion to "make a searching and fearless moral inventory." I had a hard time with the word *moral*. It felt like something I might have heard in church, before everything fell apart. As for *searching*, I thought I knew how to do that. I had searched through memories. Searched for answers to unfathomable mysteries of the past. But was I engaged in the wrong kind of search? I realized that the search I needed to do involved some basic issues about how I lived my life *in the present*. Was I good for my word? Did I tell the truth? Did I treat others the way I wanted to be treated? No, no, and no.

Step seven suggested that I "humbly" ask God to remove my short-comings. The word *humble* comes from the Latin *humus*, which means *ground*—to me that sounded perilously close to *humiliation*. The chaotic structure of my memory at the time had a way of running things together—past and present, humility and humiliation. The directive to be humble took me back to times when my mother slapped me in the face or exploded in rage; it was inconceivable to imagine that positive forward motion in life could depend on feeling that sort of low. But there are healthy ways of being in touch with the ground.

I reflected on my shortcomings. I realized how much rage and resentment I had felt, as long as I could remember. I realized how I used my pain to justify all manner of shoddy behavior through a kind of schoolyard moral calculus. I realized that if I resented someone, it was because I feared they didn't value me. But I came to recognize that I didn't have direct access to other people's minds or know what they were thinking or why they did what they did. And in any case, the inconsiderate or hurtful actions of others didn't mean I couldn't value myself. I could and should. I did not need to take the actions of others personally; their hurtful actions were the consequences of their own suffering . . . If possible, I could even attempt to seize the opportunity of witnessing these hurtful actions as a means of developing greater equanimity and compassion. However, if this was not possible, at least I could act with restraint, and only seek to regulate my own thoughts, feelings, and actions. If I felt resentful, I would have to ask what part I had played in creating the situation.

That realization laid the groundwork for step eight's suggestion that I make a list of all persons I had harmed, and be willing to make amends to them all. It was an intimidating prospect, the idea of turning backward to face the ruin of my past. The prior decade loomed in memory as a dark mass of violence, drugs, blackout drinking, psychotic visions, and suicidal thoughts, mashed together in the nonsequential and raucous form of a death-metal music video. I had an impression of my own moral agency within this miasma as a source of either guilt I could not bear or irreconcilable confusion. But Jim was a skilled guide in the backward path to the dark places. My list encompassed seventy harms in eight handwritten pages. In writing the list I discovered that the subject of more than half of those harms was—guess who—me: marijuana-induced extreme paranoia, MDMA-induced heat exhaustion in the desert, alcohol-induced blackouts and vomiting, the long depressive aftermath of drug binges. Of the other harms, the list comprised just a handful of people, hurt in the same way, over and over again—and principally Miriam.

When I was a boy at St. Peter's, I would go to confession. I went into a chamber called a confessional and confessed my sins to a priest. I remember my teacher, Mrs. Mahon, alluding in class one time to "that feeling you get after confession, when you feel so good and clean inside" in a casual way that made the feeling sound like something self-evident. I liked the sound of this good, clean feeling, but I'd never had it. "Bless me, Father, for I have sinned," I would say, but then my mind would go blank and I couldn't remember even a single misdeed I could imagine saying out loud. One time—I must have been about nine—I remembered the overdue library books that I had been afraid to tell my parents about, and how I'd enlisted my brother to help me bury them in the nearby field, and my impression of the impossibility of confessing to such a monstrous crime. I invented something that seemed more trivial instead and said my act of contrition, thinking as I prayed to God that lying in confession was surely unforgivable, and as I left the church, I tried not to think of hell. But those days were long gone.

One night I told Miriam I had something I wanted to tell her.

"I lied to you to buy drugs," I said, my voice quavering with tears. "I stole from our bank account. I yelled at you. I haven't been present for you. I'm sorry, Miriam. I'm sorry for all the ways I've hurt you. I vow never to harm you again. I can't promise I'll be perfect. But I promise to do my best."

I felt the good and clean feeling that Mrs. Mahon had mentioned all those years before and that I had never imagined would be possible for me. For the first time in my life I had an emergent understanding of the difference between two kinds of chaos in life and how I was only responsible for one of them. I didn't choose my parents. I didn't choose the family environment in which I threw my brother down the stairs. I didn't choose the chaos that traumatized me and created my vulnerability to addiction. I wasn't responsible for the path that I was born on. But my path's future direction was up to me.

My past began to feel less chaotic. I harbored no delusions of perfection. I knew I would make mistakes again. But good, bad, or indifferent, now I would do my best to learn from experience instead of running away from it.

I ONCE HEARD SOMEONE in an AA meeting say that addiction freezes your emotional development around the time you started drinking or using. Once you get sober, the person said, you pick up where you left off. That might mean you have the emotional mind of a teenager in a thirty-five-year-old body. This person was right. The available data suggest that most addicts and alcoholics start using drugs or drinking as a desperate measure to medicate the unbearable feelings associated with early life trauma. The first time a trauma survivor finds out that they can drown away bad feelings with booze or pills or powder, the discovery can feel like a miracle. *At last, something that helps! What a relief.* But once you start coping with bad feelings like this, it can be hard to stop. You don't learn other ways of coping.

I finished my first fifty-mile ultramarathon in Tahoe around the same time I finished the twelve steps. *What is my actual potential?* I wondered. I remembered paths not taken a long time before, all the way back in England when I was a teenager. *Didn't I think about becoming a doctor back then? What happened?* With a sober mind, and a stable home and family life, I could see how the chaos of my teens had derailed the opportunities I might have had at the time to contemplate different paths through life. *But what about the little boy who liked to know things? I can run fifty miles in the mountains. What else might I be able to do?* It was hard to decide what direction to go in. There were so many possibilities. Medical school seemed appealing. But once I got out, what sort of doctor could I imagine wanting to be? Psychiatry was the obvious option. But what a huge mountain I'd need to climb. I'd need to do all the premed science classes I never took in the English equivalent of high school, then get through four years of medical school and three years of residency and maybe even an additional year or two of some kind of specialized fellowship after that. If I got on it immediately, I was looking at *ten years* of school, starting in my late thirties. I figured I could do it. Nothing could ever be as hard as recovering from depression and getting sober. But at the summit of that decade-long climb, what did I imagine *actually wanting to do*? Help people the way Mike and Jim had helped me. Listen to people in pain. People like my mother and father. Like the Shopkeeper and La Llorona and Invisible Laserbeam. People like the person I once had been. The runaways.

X

Charon

Desolation Wilderness

The night is dark and cold. The sky above is black. It is early in the morning. I follow Emily down a road. The road began at the ski lodge. It was warmer back there, in the time before. It was warmer in the past. Perhaps we should have stayed there. I remember it was warm. Now the road is flat. There are pine trees on either side of us. Perhaps I should head into the trees. I could lie down on the ground. Then I would be motionless. I would like to be motionless. Then my suffering would end. I would be still among the trees. I would wait for morning. For the end of the darkness. I would see the sun again. I would sit there waiting, and then the light would come. And yet I sense this would be foolish. It is freezing here, even bundled in my coat. It is cold while I am moving. It would be colder if I stopped. I would wait and shiver. Nothing good could come of it. The darkness would last longer. The ending would not come. The ending comes to those who move toward it. Emily mentions water. Perhaps I am not drinking it. I take a sip of water. I feel it touch my lips. I swallow the cold water. It seems that she was right. I am not aware of thirst. And yet I need water. It is early and I am mourning. The night is cold and dark. The sky turns dark blue. The trail leads into the forest. Emily says eat. I listen to the doctor. I eat a GU. It hurts my mouth. My mouth has ulcers, from all the GU. I started eating them on Friday. That was days ago. Twice per hour I've had the GU, for three days straight now. Hundreds of them. It's too much GU. I don't like them. GU is nasty. Ow and yuck. Yuck and ow and yuck. I ask the doctor. I can't eat GU, I say. My mouth is hurting. My lips are hurting. My tongue is hurting. The roof of my mouth also. From all the GU. Try this, she says. It's buffalo. I eat the meat. I am not a meat eater. But I am eating it. It doesn't hurt my mouth. I eat more buffalo. Perhaps I should eat a whole one. A whole buffalo, I mean. It seems that I am moving. The sky is now light blue. Yet I still see trees around me. The end is far from here. It seems that I am moving. And yet the end is far. I am moving through the trees. It seems that I have now endured enough. And yet the trail continues. Somewhere else it is Monday morning. The ordinary world is waking up again. I was once a citizen of that distant world. My eyes are open. But I am not in any ordinary sense awake. A hundred seventy miles of mountain trail does strange things to a person. The trees ahead grow closer as the ground moves underneath me and then becomes more trees, a forest that goes on forever. Besides the trees, I am conscious of the pain. My feet hurt. My shins hurt. My shoulders and back hurt. My lips and tongue and throat hurt. Along with the pain comes the knowledge that I have chosen it and could choose to make it stop, and along with this knowledge is the understanding of the pain as an unheard cry so long blocked from awareness to which I am now willing to listen and seek to understand.

The sun rises high in the sky. I see horses in the trees. The trail leads into a clearing where there are places to sit down. "How's it going, dude?" says the medic. I tell the story of my injuries. There are others like me, she says. I meet the man to my left. His legs, like mine, are aching. He sits with his feet raised high. The Angel was here a while ago, he says. Have I met her, says the man. Yes, I tell him. In the beginning I saw the Angel. She was with me then. In the time before. "She was with us here," the man says. "The Angel came here. She tended to our suffering. I saw her. She sat with me. She has gone now. And yet long ago the Angel was once here with us. Perhaps she will return," he says. "Perhaps she will appear to us again." "We can hope for such things," I say. "How are those shins doing?" says the medic. I put my pain into words. She wraps my legs in tape. Under normal circumstances I would be skeptical that this little patch of tape could do anything for my tendons, but whether it's real or pure placebo, I'll take it.

I stand and hobble forward. "Does that feel better?" she says. "It does," I say. The tape keeps my ankles in place. The pain in my tendons reduces by a smidgen. I must rest when I reach the end, she says. There are those who return here without resting, she says. She met such a man today. He had finished another two hundred only weeks before in Washington, she says. "Dude comes in, says his foot hurt," the medic tells me. "'Take off your shoe, sir,' I said. And oh man was it gnarly. Try and run on that thing, guy, your whole heel is coming off. *Degloved* is the medical term. The flesh comes clean off the bone. 'Time for the hospital,' I told him. He went to the emergency room. Then this other guy came in, seizing. I mean full-on grand mal seizure. Some sort of electrolyte imbalance, likely. Not enough sodium or potassium. 'Get some ice over here,' I said. So he was number two for the hospital. Please don't be number three, 108!" the medic says, referring to my race number. "I promise not to," I say. "That's your number, 108?" says the man beside me. "Yes," I say. "I'm 109," he says. "What are the odds?" I calculate them. *Let* n *be 250, the set of runners. Let* x *be the chance of random selection of two consecutive bib numbers. Calculate* x. The answer proves elusive.

"Would you like some soda?" says Emily. "Yes," I say. She hands me a cup. I drink from it. Yum, cold ginger ale. I stand. I hobble forward, following Emily. The sun is lower in the sky. I am hot. My shins are hurting. The end is far; the trees surround me. The trees surround me; the end is far. I am following Emily. Oh, my shins, oh my stars, what agony with every step now! The pain becomes intolerable. "Try backward," says Emily. I try it. Going backward, my ankle flexes in the opposite direction. The pain is gone. Yet so has my velocity. I see the trail behind me, where I have been. My motions are slow and clumsy. Travel backward down the mountain and it's hard not to trip and fall.

The Enchanted Land

About a hundred miles north of San Francisco there is a twenty-five-mile stretch of pristine coastline inaccessible by roads called the Lost Coast. The closest you can get to it are the little towns at either end. Miriam and I went there a couple of years after I came to California from England. We hiked most of the trail connecting the two towns. Miriam made a watercolor painting of the view. A dark green mountain rises from the ocean in the foreground. You can see other mountains behind it, diminishing in scale, until they fade into the blue. The painting hangs above the therapy couch on my office wall.

I was twelve years sober. I had done the steps. I had made amends to the people I had hurt. I had committed to living an honest life to the best of my ability. Four years sober, I decided to go back to school. The following month I sat in a classroom for my first lecture in a clinical psychology PhD program. In class discussions or paper assignments about depression, bipolar disorder, addiction, psychosis, and other mental health issues, I felt like I was reexploring territory I'd lived for decades, and like I had an intuitive understanding for some of those far reaches of the human psyche that no amount of book learning could produce. But I also became aware of the taboo in psychology circles that discouraged clinicians from talking about their own personal or family history of mental illness. In my application essay for grad school, I'd made reference to my mother's struggles with psychosis and my own experience of depression. In my interview, I'd alluded to the letter, which I presumed the interviewer must have read. He cut me off mid-sentence, warning me that such candid disclosures would ruin my career. I was stunned. But this taboo did indeed appear to function as a central organizing principle of psychology training, reflective not so much of the institution I attended as the mental health profession as a whole: mental illness was a tragedy that happened to *other people*. We were the healers. The others were the sick ones. I heard students and even some faculty members talk routinely about "schizophrenics," "addicts," and "border-lines" like entomologists classifying insects. It made me sad. They had no idea they were talking about my parents. About La Llorona and Holst and Invisible Laserbeam and the Prisoner of Azkaban. About me. I was healthy and stable. But I had no illusions about some bright dividing line between the healthy and the sick. We are all vulnerable. In the words of Hindu guru Nisargadatta Maharaj, "There are no others."

I still felt haunted at times by familiar old feelings. Getting As, winning research awards, presenting at international conferences—for the first time in years, I was feeling like a success and that my life was going somewhere. But that sense of achievement had a shadow side. I struggled with feelings of inadequacy for which no award could compensate. I could put in a grade A performance at graduate school, but at home, Miriam and I still got into arguments that left me feeling defensive, enraged, resentful, and brooding. I'd obsess for days or even weeks over actual or perceived rejections. But when my obsessive thinking and wounded feelings got unbearable, I could always go running, and it always helped. And I signed up for about four or five ultras per year, usually with a hundred-mile run in the summer. At the time, the compulsion to keep seeking out those kinds of extreme adventures was hard for me to put into words. I wasn't consciously aware that they might offer a doorway to the feelings I was still struggling with.

I worked sixty-hour weeks for seven years to complete a doctorate in clinical psychology and two postdoctoral fellowships. I could never have imagined that the study of the mind would entail so much driving. Between the VA clinic where I saw combat veterans for trauma therapy, the hospital where I evaluated young people coping with early stage schizophrenia, the public library where I taught meditation, and the neuroimaging lab where I was researching the brain mechanisms of meditation, I sometimes drove over a hundred miles a day. One day my car broke down on the freeway, started smoking, and burst into flames. I called 911 and watched a team of first responders in special suits spray foam onto the nearby hillside, which by then was starting to smolder from the burning ruins of my Honda. I got a ride to the lab and finished an eighty-page report. There is a saying in the twelve-step world that one of the fruits of recovery is that defects become assets: after decades of chaos, a car breakdown was a bump in the road.

In the clinic, I listened to voices surrounded by the mountains. I heard voices of sorrow and despair and courage and endurance. I listened to suffering whose core wound tended to be the experience of surviving chaos that in the past had been borne alone. I saw my job as doing for others what other healers had done for me: creating an environment where people feel safe to follow the trail into the darkness. The framing perspective of the mountains in the painting reminded me where we were going: on a path toward the horizon of the known. I offered myself as a companion on that trail system of the mind. It was and remains the great honor of my life to join with others and participate in the healing that can occur when a fractured or frightened mind finds refuge within the safe horizon of an attentive consciousness. In the dead of night, it can be hard to believe that the tough spots where space and time start collapsing could ever make sense to anyone. It can feel like life has stopped in a place outside of reason. But there is a way forward. Then the trail circles round to the place you started from, but you feel safe and know the worst is behind you, that you don't need to run anymore.

ABOUT A BILLION MILES out beyond Neptune there is a ring of misshapen lumps of rock and ice called the Kuiper Belt. Pluto resides in this realm. Pluto has a moon, Charon. According to one theory, billions of years ago Pluto and Charon were a single sphere. Something massive collided into it, and they split in two. Charon stayed in orbit around Pluto, like a loyal little brother. In Greek mythology, Charon was the ferryman of the underworld. My mother mentioned him in a poem that she wrote, entitled "Enchanted Land":

> Far away from the midnight air
> A fair lady left the house.
> Somebody scribbled scrawled
> A message from the Enchanted Land.
>
> Take a boat close to the docks.
> Boatman, ferry me over the water
> Where the fairy people dwell,
> Enchanted Land away from this hell.

Like my mother, I had been in hell. I had gotten out. I knew that my mother was still suffering. She lived alone in public housing in England. She sent me emails and texts almost every day. I wrote back. I visited her with Miriam and our kids about once a year and brought her things for her flat. I wished there was more that I could do to help. I understood that I was coping with a kind of survivor's guilt. When I ran away from the ruins, I had left people behind. Mum. Dad. Sebastian. I could remember how liberating it was to escape: The feeling of the blue sky above the Black Rock Desert. The lure of a distant horizon. The blue sky feeling had stayed with me. I felt it on the trail. After years of recovery, I carried the feeling inside me. I didn't need to rush off somewhere far away again to find it. But there were other feelings I carried with me. The longer I stayed sober and built a stable life as a father, husband, runner, and psychology graduate student, the more I became aware of emotions underneath the surface of everyday awareness: the difficult feelings that before I got sober I'd have tried to suppress or distract myself from or self-medicate with drugs or alcohol. Fear. Shame. Grief. And most of all, anger: for me, that was the toughest feeling to tolerate, or even understand. I was afraid of it. Give voice to anger and I feared I might turn into my mother at her worst. But I knew I couldn't run away from feeling it, or bury it forever beneath a civilized veneer. I needed to learn how to put the feeling into words. I needed a teacher. Running is powerful medicine for the mind. But it can't heal everything.

Six years sober, I went back to therapy. I was in my third year of graduate school. Therapy is different when you're not in a state of crisis. I went deeper. I chose a psychologist trained in a kind of therapy called interpersonal psychoanalysis. His name was Dr. Carson. Interpersonal psychoanalysis was created in the 1940s by psychologist Harry Stack Sullivan. He broke with the dominant view of the talking cure that had existed since the days of Sigmund Freud and that characterized the path to understanding the mind as a journey inside the depths of an individual psyche. Sullivan believed this view was false. To understand the mind, said Sullivan, you have to understand how it formed through interactions with other minds, what he called the interpersonal field. Dr. Carson was completely different from Dr. Jensen. He didn't just sit in silence and say, *Uh-huh*, and answer a question with a question or *What would it mean to you if I answered that?* When I asked Dr. Carson a question, he told me what he thought. He shared his own thoughts and ideas about whatever I was talking about. I had no idea therapy could be like that. Lying on the couch, week after week, I began to trust that he was right behind me, paying attention to everything I said. I didn't feel like I needed to impress him. I didn't feel like he was judging me. I didn't worry that anything I wanted to share might disgust or overwhelm him. I didn't even feel like I had to make sense all the time. I could just let my mind run free, and trust that if I needed help with anything I was saying or remembering or failing to remember, I could ask him, and he would tell me what came to his mind. He didn't pretend to be omniscient. But after decades of working with people who had survived traumatic early life experiences, he had some solid ideas about the nature of human development and the ways that early trauma shapes a growing mind. "I see my job as helping people understand feelings they have about experiences they lived through but can't remember," he said. "I want you to know that you're supposed to have *all* your feelings. I want you to be okay with experiencing your anger, and talking about it."

I came to understand why it had taken me so long to make sense of my past, circling back on the same shards of memory, again and again, but never feeling as if I touched the core of whatever it was I'd been through.

In the presence of Dr. Carson, I reflected on my collapse into the Darkness when I was fifteen. How apocalyptic that moment had seemed. It hadn't made sense at the time. With the passage of years, it made even less sense, looking back. How could two mediocre exam results feel like the end of the world? Between my unbearable feelings and the memory of the experience that appeared to evoke them, there was a gap. A void.

I reflected on other voids. The day I lay on my bed in uncontrollable tears after I hid the candy in my boots. The day I ran down the mountain. My dread of nuclear holocaust. The inexplicable sadness that followed me around India. Each time I fled the Darkness, I didn't look back. I felt like I was running away. But I was following an unconscious path that led me around in a circle, back into the same feelings of fear and rage and despair.

I reflected on my earliest memories and stories of experiences I lived through prior to conscious memory. The day my mother left me in the van. I wondered about even earlier experiences, times perhaps as an infant when I was alone and frightened in the dark and no one heard my cry.

Sometimes late at night, running in the mountains, seventy or eighty miles into a hundred-mile run, a feeling of depletion would seep through my soul that reminded me of the hell I had suffered in my downward slide toward the psychic death of severe depression. One of those nights I found myself walking slowly on a snowy trail thousands of feet above Lake Tahoe. I had been awake and moving through the mountains for twenty hours. There had been record snowfall in the Sierra Nevada. I shivered in the cold. I shuffled forward on bandaged feet, wincing with pain from blisters. I couldn't remember why I had ever set forth on such a futile and arbitrary ritual of self-punishment. *I'm done*, I thought. *At the next aid station, I'm bailing.* My mind was made up. As the aid station got closer, I announced my decision to my pacer, a veteran ultrarunner by the name of Rajeev. He tried to talk me out of quitting. "But it's only twenty miles to go!" he said. "You're so close! You can do it!" He tried telling me stories of ultrarunners plumbing similar depths of overwhelm and dejection and finding their way forward to redemption in the dawn. He recited verse by the Indian poet Ghalib. I was long past the persuasive reach of positivity, via verse or fable. All I could think about was getting into a hot bath and seeing Miriam. I hobbled down the mountain to a ski lodge near the lake. I took off my race bib and got a ride to my lodgings. I had my hot bath and went to bed. Miriam had gone out somewhere. Following a couple of hours of dreamless sleep I awoke with feelings of despair and thoughts that I had failed in some profound way. The intensity of those feelings seemed disproportionate even at the time to the ostensible fact of an unfinished mountain run. I felt like an unfinished person. In the results on ultrarunning websites the acronym for those who do not finish is DNF: did not finish. I had finished plenty of ultras in the past. I could finish plenty more in the future, if I chose to do so. *But will that take away this unfinished feeling? Or am I a spiritual DNF?*

My life in many respects remained a stable one. I loved being a dad. I loved being married to Miriam, building a life and family together. And I loved graduate school. I loved learning how to listen and respond with care and skill to patients in psychotherapy, integrating everything I had learned about the body and the mind from books and hard-won life experience. And I loved exploring deep scientific questions about the neurology of self-awareness. To me those questions weren't abstract: they were matters of life and death.

But the unfinished feeling stayed with me. A vague sense of lack. Being in graduate school certainly compounded that perception. Psychology training was like a mountain with a hundred false summits before you reach the actual peak. I was always applying for something. A position in a research lab. A clinical placement. An internship. Then a postdoctoral fellowship. Then *another* postdoctoral fellowship: You know, just because.

Because I could never be smart enough. Good enough. Because *I* was never enough. On an emotional level, I hadn't moved on from who I was in Mrs. Mahon's class at St. Peter's Primary School, the little boy with all the right answers.

And there were things I still didn't know, a kind of knowledge that I sensed I wouldn't acquire no matter how many fancy fellowships I pursued: the kind of insights that bubbled up as if from nowhere in a long run, when the thinking mind shuts down, beyond the threshold of reason.

One day I was sitting in the office, on a break between patients. I had finished seven years of clinical training, passed the state and national exams for licensure as a psychologist, and gotten a job as a psychotherapist in a community clinic in a high-poverty neighborhood in the Bay Area. Scrolling through an ultrarunning website, looking for my next adventure, I came across a listing for the Tahoe 200. As I pictured the lake in the mountains, a memory of meeting Miriam there almost twenty years before flashed into my mind. Then I remembered my first fifty-mile ultramarathon on the Tahoe Rim Trail, and the transformative moment in that run that propelled me on the forward path that sent me running another ten thousand miles toward the life I now had as a happy father and husband and psychologist. I wondered what might happen if I went back there.

I sensed that it might be time to look back again. I hadn't done so in a while. After I had finished the twelve steps, the following decade had been all about moving forward. Sobriety frees up an astounding amount of energetic bandwidth. Between taking my kids to school, cooking, cleaning, reading bedtime stories, cramming for exams, sitting with patients in session, writing academic papers, traveling to conferences, and running trails, every day was a sort of multidisciplinary ultramarathon. Meanwhile Miriam was working just as hard, if not harder, as a parent and in her work as an industrial designer. By the time we curled up together in bed at night for a few minutes of Netflix before we zonked out, my heart was full of gratitude. But days as full as that didn't leave much time for looking back at the steps that led up to the present, to make sense of the shape of the trail. The view from where I was in the present, looking forward a couple of steps, was more than enough.

But that day, seeing a photo of the lake on my computer screen, I reflected on the long path I'd traveled from the chaos of my teenage years in England, through the psych ward and AA meetings to the neuroscience lab and the clinic I was sitting in, waiting for my next patient to arrive. I was conscious of having reached firm ground after traveling an improbable path. My recovery from depression and addiction was never guaranteed—there were many times when I had come close to death by suicide or drug overdose—but I was more fortunate than some. I found it illuminating to consider how even slight variations in that path might have led me into permanent darkness. Swap Mrs. Mahon for someone less caring and I might never have embraced books and reading in the way that got me into Oxford and in the end my doctorate. Cancel my trip to Burning Man in 1999 and I'd never have met Miriam. Remove Dr. Jensen, Dr. Browning, Dr. Hewitt, or Mike, and I might never have gotten out of that bathtub. Swap white skin for black or brown skin when the police stopped me while driving high and I might well have wound up in prison or shot to death. Take away Jim and AA and I'd likely have relapsed on cocaine and wound up divorced and miserable or buried in a box underground. Take away Dr. Carson and I never would have understood the painful feelings that lingered from experiences I'd lived through but could only recall in fragments or not at all. Take away the mountain trails and I never would have felt the joy in early recovery that showed me life could be worth living, that provided the strength to explore new paths, and that gave me a space to dream.

What a long, strange trip it had been. It occurred to me that someone, somewhere, might feel encouraged by hearing what I'd been through. I had no illusion that my experience was universal. And I was aware that mental health professionals almost never tell their own stories. Nothing in the law or the ethical codes of the mental health professions prohibits clinician self-disclosure. It is an unspoken, informal convention that nonetheless functions with a lawlike force, restraining candid speech.

The conventional wisdom used to be that in order for therapy to work, therapists needed to function as "blank slates" upon which patients could project their longings, needs, and fantasies without the interference of knowing their therapists' actual biographies. But the blank slate is a myth: therapists can't avoid disclosing aspects of their identities automatically, for no other reason than their existence is embodied in directly observable features like ethnicity or age. Yet the de facto prohibition against therapist self-disclosure persists, in large part I believe because of stigma, and perhaps an overidentification by therapists in a "helper" role and corresponding anxieties around any concessions to their own experiences of human vulnerability. I believe it's time as a society that we move forward to a more honest and open dialogue about the reality of mental health. Removing stigma won't eliminate mental illness, but it will make it easier to talk about it without adding an extra dose of shame to an already painful experience. Nobody wants the therapist who responds to the patient's story by saying, "Well, you think *you've* got problems . . ." The point of therapy is to heal the patient, not the doctor. But I don't believe that any harm can come from greater clinician self-disclosure within appropriate circumstances. To the contrary, perhaps clinicians could model a compassionate and nonjudgmental attitude about mental illness by giving voice to their own experiences.

I stared at the lake on my computer screen, and I contemplated the prospect of running nonstop for days and nights the whole way around it, and I tried to picture just how exhausted I might become in the ultramarathon's later miles, and whether I was brave enough to submit to such an ordeal, and what sort of lessons I might learn once I spent long enough in the waking dreamworld of the mountain run, once I reached the limits of reason, and stepped beyond them.

..

It's around eight in the evening, Monday. My fourth straight day in the mountains. The trail's winding downhill in the twilight. I've been on my feet and moving for seventy-two of the past eighty hours. Everything has hurt too much, for too long, wearing me down. I'm ready to drop. I don't think anyone could hold it against me. I've run one hundred eighty miles. Climbed around thirty thousand feet of rugged mountain trail. Struggled through heat and cold and dizziness for four days and three nights on just eight hours sleep in total. The end is still twenty-four miles away, over the hardest section of the course, an extremely steep, boulder-strewn jeep track called the Rubicon Trail, followed by a two-thousand-foot climb to Barker Pass, followed by a seven-mile descent to complete the clockwise circle back at Homewood. The final cutoff for runners to complete the race is noon tomorrow. That gives me twelve hours to cover twenty-four steep, rough miles. Moving at my current glacial pace, to have any hope at all of covering the distance still ahead in the time available, I'll need to nix my catnap and plod the whole night through. It's a nightmarish prospect. No doubt if I drop now I'll feel a twinge of disappointment tomorrow. But I'll take it. At least I can stop soon. There's only so much suffering I can bear.

The trail takes me out of the trees and into a backcountry parking lot. I hear Miriam cheering before I see her beaming face.

"I'm done," I say. "It's too hard. I can't do it. I'm bailing."

Miriam shakes her head. She's all kitted out in her running clothes, headlamp, backpack, and trekking poles, ready to pace me to the end like we'd planned.

"There is absolutely no way you are not finishing this thing!" she says, with the kind of joyful exuberance that made me fall in love with her. Some fires are so warm and toasty, you never want to put them out. How could I let her down?

"Okay," I say. I sit down. I change my shoes and socks. I ask a medic to patch up my blisters. I say goodbye to Emily and Andrew and kiss the kids goodbye. They'll stay with Emily and Andrew tonight, who'll take them to school tomorrow morning. Then Miriam leads me into the darkness. I follow her on a dusty trail heading uphill. It's all I can do to put one foot in front of the other. I hear Miriam talking, catching me up on her day with the kids. I can't focus on what she's saying. It's not the topic that I'm having a hard time managing to process but language itself. My thinking mind is shutting down altogether. My brain's working at something like the level of a three-year-old. *Are we there yet? I don't like this. I wanna go home . . .*

XI

Dysnomia

The Tower

Out beyond the Kuiper Belt there is an even more distant realm of icy rocks called the Scattered Disc. One of them is called Dysnomia, named after the Greek god of anarchy. There is a school of thought that anarchy never accomplishes anything worthwhile. But chaos can be creative, the seed of breakthrough, rather than breakdown.

Kazimierz Dąbrowski was a twentieth-century Polish psychiatrist. When he was in his twenties, his best friend died by suicide. When he was in his forties, the Nazis put him in prison. After World War II, Stalin put him in prison again. Dąbrowski sought to understand an apparent paradox about the chaos of war: its capacity to yield both heroism and murder, the best and worst poles of human behavior. He developed a theory he called *positive disintegration*.[15] Psychological maturity requires the ability to see life from what Dąbrowski called a multileveled perspective. An immature person sees the world from a rigid, single point of view: me versus you, us versus them. A mature person sees the world from a flexible point of view, moving between different perspectives and integrating them. To shift from a rigid, all-or-nothing, single-level state to a flexible, multilevel state, a certain kind of creative chaos—positive disintegration—is necessary. Disintegration doesn't always end well. It can be negative, as Dąbrowski witnessed in his friend's suicide and the atrocities of Hitler and Stalin. But chaos can be harnessed toward transformational ends.

Recent neuroscience research has illuminated some of the brain mechanisms involved in positive disintegration. The principal breakthroughs in this area have come from research on the clinical use of psychedelic drugs. The use of psilocybin for depression and anxiety in cancer patients suggests that the therapeutic benefits involve the stimulation of a disordered brain state similar to a waking dream. Neuroscientist Robin Carhart-Harris calls this state the *entropic brain*.[16] Psychedelics induce a waking dream by increasing the amount of entropy, or disorder, in the network structure of the brain. Under ordinary circumstances the brain maintains a balance between two essential modes of consciousness, primary and secondary. Primary consciousness is the mind of emotion and dreams and infant reverie. Secondary consciousness is the mind of thought and reason. The brain is a system of electrochemical circuits negotiating a balance between order and disorder. Psychedelics push the balance toward disorder. It is this chaotic state, Carhart-Harris proposes, that can reorganize the rigid neural patterns associated with anxiety and depression.

Can ultrarunning, like psychedelic drugs, induce the entropic brain? Proof awaits confirmation through empirical studies. Eighty-four hours into the Tahoe 200, I sure *felt* like I was tripping on acid—though for a while not in a positive way. I was in Dysnomia: a state of psychological anarchy, on the verge of breakdown.

WORDS. THERE ARE MANY of them, these words, running together, one upon the other. Long ago I might have known their meaning. I might have heard about a river. Children. A boat upon the river. Children. Boat. River. I would have heard these words and turned them into pictures in my mind. I would have seen the children on the river. She is telling me about the time before. The old time, before I came here. Now there are boulders in every direction. A rock. Step over it. Another rock. Step over it. More rocks, forever. Focus on the next ten steps. Get from here to that bush over there. One. Throbbing pain, from ankle to knee. Accept it. You can do this. Two. Stabbing pain. Three. Another stab. You can do it. Breathe. Four. Stab. Five. Stab. Six. Stab. Stop. Kneel down. Sit on your heels. Stretch out the shins. No pain now. I could stay here, kneeling. Then the pain would disappear. I could kneel and pray for morning. But then the end would never come. I see two men by the side of the trail ahead of me. One man is lying down. The other sits by him, waiting. Perhaps they were promised the morning, these men. Perhaps they know something that I do not. One . . . two . . . three. I pass the men. The trail leads to the edge of a vast, steep plunge into nothingness. I can't see the ground beneath the shroud of dust that covers it. I take a slow step forward. A jagged rock stabs my feet. I look at the path ahead. The boulder maze extends as far as I can see. The world's shrunk to a pale sphere of light beyond whose frontiers the forest disappears into the void. I can smell the stink that wafts from a body encrusted with days of sweat. I feel dizzy from fatigue and lack of oxygen at this high altitude. Pain from my blistered feet cuts like a dagger with each—*Ow!*—step—*Ow!*—forward. My legs throb in agony after days and nights of running over almost two hundred miles of rugged mountain trail. I have nothing left to give. But I can't stop. The end is fifteen miles from here—it might as well be a billion. I know that all I can and must do is take—this—next—step. At least the ground is flat. It's the descents that punish my aching shin tendons. I take—another—step. A maze of jagged boulders. The air thick with dust. A patch of ground lit by the sick yellow rays of my headlamp. A shroud of dust flattens the ground from three dimensions into two. Behold the collapse of space. The darkness seems infinite, severing the moment from past and future, stranding me here alone in pain. Behold the collapse of time. Perhaps I am supposed to be here, alone and hurting, in the darkness beyond all reason. I am back in the dark place. Rocks plunge into an abyss. A flat plane ahead. One. Another rock dagger. The mountain hates me. One, two, three. Stab, stab, stab. I must have done something very bad. The trail descends farther into the void. One . . . two . . . three. Kneel again. No pain. Then the knowledge of the distance still ahead. Standing, moving, the right and then the left. Rocks everywhere. The mountain smashed into pieces. Pain in my toes, pain in my shins, pain in my mouth and mind. What's in your boots? Blisters. The need to keep on running. The need to remember something.

Right foot. Left foot. Right foot, left foot. *You've really gone downhill, wee fella.* Right foot. Left foot. Right foot. Dark. Dark. Dark. The sun has died. Breathe in. Breathe out. Plant the left pole. Now the right one. *Hear the clock tick-tock. Hear the children play by the river. You may hear tones and then silence.* One, two, left, right. *You may hear moans and then silence.* Right, stab. Left, stab. You are at the lowest level. There is no boulder beneath this one. *Moans. Silence.* Plant the left pole. Now the right one. *Hear the children moan by the river. English male, disheveled, welcome to the City of Night.* Another. Step. Forward. One. One. One. *Ouch. Ouch. Ouch.* Breathe in. Breathe out. Dust in the air, dust on the ground. Kneel again. No pain. Then standing and moving and the pain again. *The patient understands the rule. Dot, dot, dot. Right? You could have gone anywhere. You came here.* The clock. Tick. Stops. One, two, three. Ashes in the air, ashes on the ground. *Daddy, please save me from the Bomb.* I cannot remember the explosion. Oblivion. One, two, three. *Trap shut, gob shut. Trap shut, gob shut. Ball, book, flag. Repeat after me: if I get lost or die, it's my own damn fault. I am lost and dead. My fault. Mummy is lost and dead. My fault.* I remember everything and nothing. One. Two. Three. *Ball. Book. Flag.* One. Two. Three. Left. Right. Left. *Tell me the three things I asked you to remember. Mum. Is. Dead. Mother is dead. The others are dead. Repeat after me: shut up, shut up, shut up. Clean your teeth and shut your mouth. The runner understands the rules.* The trees say, *Hello, wake up. Wake up, wake up, wake up. Hear the clock tick-tock, hear the ghosts and silence. Ball. Book. Oblivion.* Dust in the air . . . dust in my eyes and nose . . . ashes in my eyes. *I can't breathe. I can't think. Help . . .*

A LIGHT COMES ON in the depths of my scattered consciousness. *I'm not alone and lost and helpless in an infinite darkness. I'm here in the mountains, with Miriam. I know what to do.* "I have to sleep," I say. "Immediately." "Sure, babe," says Miriam. I stride to the side of the trail and hurl myself to the ground on a pile of pine needles. I take off my pack and pull out my survival blanket. I wrap the golden foil around me. Miriam lies down next to me and gets underneath the blanket. I close my eyes, cocooned in my blanket and Miriam's arms. A maelstrom of dream images rushes through my mind.

My eyes open. Ten minutes have passed. I am restored to lucid waking awareness. I stand. There's a way out of here: one step at a time. The sun will rise, the darkness will end, and I'll get back to Homewood. I follow Miriam downhill for a little while longer until we reach the bottom of the boulder maze. The trail ahead is a steep slog two thousand feet up to the last aid station before the finish. Barker Pass: mile 198.5. Miriam sets a solid pace on the climb. I can see her in my headlamp about thirty feet ahead. I catch up with another runner. "Top five, top three hardest things you've ever done?" he says. "No question," I say. The two of us fall into a rhythm, matching each other step for step, until we reach the final summit. Inside the tent at Barker Pass I can see cots and blankets and a heater and tables loaded with food. I can see an exhausted runner, collapsed on a cot. I grab a plate of food and sit down by one of the heaters. I sit facing a man bundled up in blankets. I listen to him speaking to the woman sitting next to him, whom I recognize as the medic who tended to my injuries a long time ago.

"And we do this—for what?" says the man. "For a medal? A shirt? So that we can say *we were there*? Why do we do these things?" It was hard to know. He could have been a prophet, gazing down with sad eyes at the folly of the world. You could sit on a mountaintop and ask questions like that until the end of time.

A little while before I went to the hospital, when I was obsessing over what happened in Cannon Road, my father consulted the I Ching, the ancient Chinese book of spiritual prophecy. My father interpreted the text he read through this consultation with the following guidance to me: "It is as though you have climbed a high tower. From the top, you can see farther. But you can only see as far as the horizon. You must come down from the tower. When you do, you will gain the power to change a number of people's lives."

I DIDN'T COME DOWN from the tower for many years. It was so lonely up there, I almost died. I kept looking at the view. I gazed at every single tree. The past is infinite. The more you look at it, the more you understand. There's no end to understanding. But now I understand enough. I've seen the trees. I won't forget them. I've looked at the view so long, I can close my eyes and still see the forest. I'll never forget it. The forest is a part of me. So now it's finally time to go. I'm ready. It's time to come down from the tower. It's time to try and change a number of people's lives. Even if that number is one.

"Let's get out of here," I say.

"Good call," says Miriam. "This place is freaking me out."

We hike out of Barker Pass at about two in the morning and start a long descent following the last seven miles of the trail as it circles back to Homewood. When the sun comes up, I can see the lake. We head downhill for hours, but it feels like the lake's not gotten any closer, as if the circle around the lake has formed a kind of magic island that I will never leave.

Around nine in the morning I can hear claps and whoops from the crowd at the finish line. A bell rings. It's hard to believe that soon I'll sit down and won't need to run anymore.

XII

The Oort Cloud

Stay Awhile

I hobbled along the busy downtown street in a dreamy state of mind. I was on my way to the courthouse. My legs still hurt. My mind was still reeling from ninety-six hours of running. I was due in court to testify as an expert witness in an asylum case. One of the patients at our clinic was a young man from Guatemala. He'd fled gang violence there and sought sanctuary in California. He'd survived a kind of violence on a scale altogether different from the challenges I endured in my own youth as a white man growing up in England. But I could empathize with the impetus of a fellow runaway seeking refuge someplace far away. As I made my way to the court, a crowd flowed past me. Everyone looked like they were in a rush to get where they were going, heads downcast to the sidewalk or a phone, no one looking forward or at the cloudless sky above. I wanted to high-five every one of them as if they were fellow travelers on the trail of life, saying, *Good job, friend—you got this*. My body had come back to the city. But my mind was still in the mountains, chanting, *Namu kie Butsu*. Perhaps it always would be.

The dreamy feeling stayed with me. It took a while to process what had happened on my last night in Tahoe. The meaning revealed itself in hindsight, like the route up a dark mountain I had only glimpsed in disconnected little parts at the time as I took each step uphill but that I could see as whole in the sunrise at the summit, looking back downhill. For so long I had wondered about all the holes in my memory, all the voids in my history, a vague intuition of something incomplete and forever mysterious and irrecoverable in my sense of who I was, where I came from, the throb of an ancient wound. *What happened in Cannon Road? What happened to my parents? Why did the model and the soldier run away?*

They were the wrong questions. I had been searching for answers in the past, in memory or history. But the knowledge I'd lost wasn't there. It didn't exist in time at all. Ninety hours into the run, at the point the waking dream became nightmarish, something felt all too familiar. The mountain was massive and terrifying. The darkness was infinite. I felt alone. I understood the infinite darkness as a time outside of time, when I was little and helpless and afraid. I was all by myself in the presence of something massive and incomprehensible: my mother's psychosis. But now I understood her mind, and my own. I wouldn't need to go back into the darkness ever again. This was what I learned in the fourth night in the mountains, running around the lake. This was the knowledge in the shadows.

I felt as if I had woken from a long and crazy dream. I could picture the early miles in the sunshine, high above the lake. The endless marching through the green tunnel of the forest. Infinite corridors of darkness, slogging up mountains in the night. The Mourner and Kindness and Mountain Buddha. The sensation of the whole of my past, the long trail from England to the present, folded inside the inner space that opened up and widened as I traveled farther outward. I had wanted to find the message that lay deep in the shadows. On the fourth night, I had found it. The meaning emerged in my mind over several months, as I followed the trail of memory from the nightmare world of the fourth night in Tahoe back into the past. Suicide. Drugs. Time after time, I stood at the edge of the abyss. I kept on circling back to the time it had always been, the place where I had stopped. There were parts of me I still didn't understand. Voids in time that no amount of thinking or remembering or studying could ever fill in. But on the fourth night in Tahoe, I had finally traveled to that dream-world with the knowledge preserved upon waking of what and whom my dream self had encountered there. I'd gone to Tahoe because of an intuition operating at the most primordial level of my mind, the way we experience the world as infants and in other liminal states of consciousness like dreams. This level precedes rational thought and has its own rules that function according to a kind of magical illogic. If this unconscious part of me could speak, it would have expressed a belief as follows: *If I collapse, Mummy will come back to me.* Once there was a frightened little boy alone in his room. Then there was a man in the hospital, remembering the boy in the room. Then a runner on a mountain, remembering the man in the hospital, remembering the boy in the room. The mountain and the rooms were one. I kept collapsing, trying to stay connected to her, or to the place we shared where our minds ran into each other. But I didn't need to do that anymore.

I told Shosan what I had learned. Several months later I participated in the *jukai* ceremony, where I committed to the vows of Zen Buddhism. It was a fitting acknowledgment of the long trail that led from the present moment back through the mountains that had healed me, to the hospital, to the Black Rock Desert, to England, Ireland, back through space and time. "All of my ancient twisted karma, from beginningless greed, hatred, and delusion, born through body, speech, and mind, I now fully avow," I said three times, following Zen tradition for the ceremony. At the end of the ceremony, Shosan gave me a new name: Yakuzan. It means Medicine Mountain.

SIX MONTHS AFTER I got back from Tahoe my brother sent me a text asking when I had last heard from our mother. I checked my phone. Two weeks had passed since her last text. The silence was unusual. She was a prolific texter. I made some phone calls. I tracked her down in a public hospital. She had fallen. She had lain on the ground for two days. She was found when a neighbor heard her banging her shoe against the radiator. Why she had lain there all that time was something of a mystery. In the public housing unit where she lived, the social services had installed an emergency cord for frail seniors to pull in an emergency to summon help. Mum had been lying right underneath the cord. She surely could have reached to grab it if she'd wanted to. Like so many other falls in our family across the generations, this one was a mystery.

I got on a plane to England. She looked frail and much thinner than the last time I had seen her. She must have weighed a hundred pounds. She smiled when she saw me entering the ward. I sat down by her bed.

"What happened?" I said.

"I fell," she said. She couldn't remember the moment of the fall. Why she lay on the ground all that time, she couldn't say.

We were silent for a while. I told her that I had driven past our old house earlier that day. I could remember our lovely garden, I said.

"Yes," she said. "Apples. Peas. Potatoes. Roses. Lavender blooming."

I could remember visiting Ireland in our summer holidays, I said. I could remember the beach and the sea and the mountains. I could remember a farm we visited nearby. "I think you went there as a girl," I said.

"Yes," she said. "There was a river. And stepping-stones. We played in the river. It was very deep—I was very little."

"You used to sing," I said.

"Yes," she said. "I won six medals."

"You were a dancer," I said.

"Yes," she said. "Irish dancing."

"Hard," I said.

"Yes. Very hard."

"You would climb the mountains," I said.

"Yes," she said.

"I remember the day we climbed Slieve Donard and I ran down without you," I said. "Do you remember what happened? I always thought you must have been angry with me. Can you remember why I ran away?"

She shook her head. "You probably wanted to be first," she said. "First down the mountain."

We were silent for a while again before resuming our reminiscence. As we spoke, I was conscious of a trail that seemed to form between our two minds that traveled back through time to a life we had once shared. I could remember how I had once needed to run away in fear of a mind I did not understand. I was conscious of sitting close to her now, and how, as I held her in my attention, she seemed to be present in one moment and then absent in the next, like a mind that circled between daytime and the night.

Time passed. I stood to leave.

"Are you going now?" she said.

"Yes," I said. "But I'm coming back tomorrow. Good night. I love you."

AT THE FARTHEST REACHES of the solar system some astronomers say there's a ring of distant objects called the Oort Cloud. The objects number in the tens of thousands, a ring of misshapen frigid lumps, wandering their lonely course over the hundred thousand years it takes them to complete a single orbit of the sun. The gravitational force of the sun extends outward in a zone called a Hill sphere. The objects at the outer frontier of the Oort Cloud lie at the very edge of the sun's Hill sphere—perhaps a light-year from the sun: six trillion miles. From out here the sun looks nothing like the warm, friendly yellow circle you can see from here on Earth. From a perspective exiled way out in the Oort Cloud, the sun shrinks to a point of light in the firmament, as Arcturus or Rigel appears to us on Earth. At the limits of the sun's gravitational force, objects in the Oort Cloud sometimes spin off into interstellar space.

There is an Oort Cloud of lost human possibility. This is the space that enfolds the runaways that disappeared: lives cut short by trauma, violence, addiction, or suicide. Their lives were incomplete. They lived with pain that became unendurable. They never came to experience the lives that might have existed for them. This space also contains frozen distant objects at the far frontiers of the unconscious mind: parts of our self and our history so painful we've pushed them to the very outer orbit of the light of consciousness, our deepest shame, sadness, regret. The force that binds these broken parts of us is so weak, sometimes they split off from us altogether and wander into the spaces beyond. These lost souls, these abandoned parts of the self, now reside in a virtual zone, a distant circle of being that persists like the Oort Cloud at the far frontier of awareness, barely still contained within the orbit of consciousness. Some of their names are known to us as people we once knew alive. Others are unknown, unmourned, forgotten. The task of honoring the unlived potential of those whose names are remembered, imagining the potential of those names whom history passed over in darkness, and acknowledging the parts of our individual and collective histories that we have denied or forgotten falls to those of us still living.

IN THE MORNING, I went to my mother's flat to organize her belongings. In the kitchen, I saw some photos taped to the fridge. One of them was a black-and-white image of some schoolgirls. I recognized my mother, seated in the middle of the group. She looked about ten. She's all dressed up in her smart shirt and blazer, beaming with pride. I wondered what kind of life she had dreamed of back then. I could see such hope in her smiling face. Perhaps she knew nothing yet about the soldier and the model. But perhaps she did know and the discovery didn't trouble her, when there was so much else to think about. Dances. Singing competitions. The infinite possibility of the future, the way it seems to a ten-year-old, stretching ahead to a far horizon across a vast and spacious land. I wondered if the story of the soldier and the model, her original parents, the ones who ran away, was the way she began to make sense of herself when she was older, looking back at the voids in history, and then at the void within, the parts of her own mind that transcended comprehension, her scattered thoughts and frantic feelings, the runaway parts that refused to cohere in any kind of meaning, and then understood the two mysteries as one, as if the possibility of ever feeling whole again ran away with her parents across the sea.

Another photo depicted Sebastian and me with our mother near the summit of Slieve Donard when I was ten. It occurred to me that the photo must have been taken on the day when I ran down the mountain. But the little boy in the picture was smiling. The look on his happy face reminded me of a certain cute expression I loved to see on my nine-year-old son. I wondered about the hole in my memory of that day, the space I had filled for so long with the thought that I must have been angry or afraid. It seemed hard to believe that the happy boy in the picture could have felt such inner turmoil. *There was joy before the fear. There was light in the time before the darkness came. There was light inside the darkness in the beginning and through all of time.*

In the closet there was an old teddy bear. He had the august and threadbare look of a beloved childhood companion. From the bed—I could see from the angle—my mother would have been able to see him, seated several feet above her in the closet. I could picture her alone in the nighttime, feeling the imaginary comfort of this old friend, the lovely old bear who watched over her. I wondered if she could still see him after her fall. I could imagine her collapsed on the floor, with a toy bear as her only friend in the universe. I felt a great wave of grief, absorbing the knowledge of how long she must have suffered such isolation.

In the back of the closet there were some battered black leather briefcases. The briefcases were stuffed full of old bills and junk mail. Sorting through the papers, I found some notebooks. They were full of her poems. She must have written hundreds. There were dates underneath the poems. They went back years. Cannon Road was in them. England in the wintertime. The Irish mountains in the summer. Her two little boys. Her son, a doctor in the family. One of the poems read as follows:

First
Kiss
Not
Forgotten

Stay
Awhile
Remember
Happy
Childhood

Childhood ends. But you never forget your first kiss. Childhood's joy and wonder is always present, if you look for it, in the wild places, the forest of the mind.

I couldn't reverse what had happened to my family in the '80s. I couldn't rebuild my childhood home in my mind. I had to lay the past to rest. But letting go of the past didn't mean running away from it. It meant learning from the lessons of history: understanding the knowledge in the shadows.

IT WAS A WARM summer's day when I returned to visit my mother again a few months later. Following her long rehab, she'd moved to a nicer flat with more support from social services. She had made only minimal progress in physiotherapy. She was confined to a chair, immobilized, shuffling to the toilet with a walker and the aid of the caregivers who visited four times each day. She had given up. I offered her my hands. She stood. She walked in slow steps, holding my hands for balance. We went outside into a grassy courtyard in whose center stood an oak. We walked in a circle around the tree and then settled on a bench. I could see she was out of breath. "How do you feel?" I said. "Exhilarated!" she said. "Like my feet are coming alive."

..

The vast blue lake looks so close now I could almost leap right into it. The finish can't be more than a quarter-mile away. On a morning like this, running down the mountain, crying happy tears, my mind runs wild.

Anything seems possible. I can imagine a run that never ends, on a circle going all the way around the world, on a sunny day when every child comes skipping from the schoolhouse, when madmen run laughing on the rooftops, when every prisoner runs from liberty to redemption, when every river runs with clear, clean water, when deer leap through living forests that stretch to every horizon, when every runaway finds home.

ACKNOWLEDGMENTS

The visionary mid-twentieth-century English psychoanalyst Wilfred Bion believed that a new mother "dreams" her baby's mind into existence: the self first forms in an intersubjective realm, an imaginary space in which parent and infant are one. The story in this book is mine. But in writing it, I was never alone. Many wise minds helped dream these pages into being.

I bow down to my ancestors and to all my teachers. I thank great teacher Shakyamuni, Bodhidharma, Eihei Dogen, Shunryu Suzuki Roshi, Shosan Gigen, and all of my brothers and sisters on the path of liberation.

I offer my deep respect and gratitude to the native peoples upon whose ancestral lands I have been fortunate to run: the Ohlone, the Coastal Miwok, and the Washoe.

Thank you, runners, for your company on the trail. Special thanks to the Saturday Morning Tam Runners, the San Quentin Thousand Mile Club, and to Candice Burt and Angel Mathis and everyone at Destination Trail.

I am grateful for all the teachers and fellow writers, beginning in primary school and continuing into my adulthood, who introduced me to the magical world of books and literature, and who taught me how to read, write, and think. Thanks to my Oxford University tutors, Nicola Trott, Seamus Perry, and Philip Wheatley. Thanks to Steven Poole, Rupert Brow, Renee Swindle, Rebecca Wilson, Geoff Dyer, Larry Smith, and Josh Davis, for encouraging me during my long genesis as a writer.

Thanks to Bonnie Nadell and Austen Rachlis at Hill Nadell Literary, for believing in this book from the moment I met you: I appreciate your patience, insight, and professionalism. Thanks to Gideon Weil, Sydney Rogers, and everyone involved with this book at HarperOne. I could not have hoped for a more skillful editorial team: in working with you as I delivered drafts and then a final manuscript, I felt like a nervous parent, passing a firstborn child into the warm hands of a trustworthy extended family.

Three close friends provided astute feedback to drafts. Thanks to Debbie Berne and Aran Watson. Special thanks to Ben Lewis: psychiatrist, ultrarunner, and scholar of philosophy (is there anyone else on Earth more uniquely qualified to comment on this book, or gab together for hours about neuroscience and Zen in some faraway desert or canyon?). I am lucky to know you and your lovely family.

I am forever indebted to my healers: the mental health professionals who saved my life. I do not name them in these pages, because to do so might complicate their relationship with their current patients. I am thankful too for the fellowship and solidarity of peers in recovery, whose anonymity I have likewise preserved.

In my own subsequent training as a psychologist, I have benefited from the mentorship and guidance of many gifted clinicians, researchers, scholars, supervisors, and colleagues in the health professions and other fields. Thank you to Steve Hinshaw for inspiring me with the notion that I could become a psychologist because of—rather than despite—my challenging prior personal history. Thank you to Willi McFarland, Anu Banerjee, John Sadler, Peter Zachar, Rebecca Gitlin, Jeannie Celestial, Sandra Macias, Joyce Chu, the late Nigel Field, Janice Habarth, Lynn Waelde, Rowena Gomez, Jarred Younger, David Spiegel, Fletcher Thompson, Helen Hsu, Maria St. John, Allison Briscoe-Smith, Barbara Stuart, Daniel Mathalon, Anda Kuo, Tom Boyce, Nicki Bush, Danielle Rubinov, Rick Hecht, Eve Ekman, Dean Schillinger, Shannon Wozniak, JayVon Muhammad, Karuna Leary, Dominique McDowell, Brooke Lavelle, and Jeff Duncan-Andrade.

Thank you to the hundreds of individuals in whose healing I have been honored in recent years to participate through my work as a psychotherapist: it has been a privilege to walk the trail of transformation with you.

Thank you to my friends. Trauma is a disease of loneliness—but you never gave up on me. I would like to acknowledge, in particular, Steve Rolles and the Rolles family, Lucy Platt, Nick Lockley, Gavin Rees, Edward Purver, Robin Batt, Victoria Coren Mitchell, Charlie Skelton, Tom Hooper, Peter Sweasey, Daniel Fugallo, Roy Ackerman, Ursula Macfarlane, Batul Mukhtiar, Lenny Oliker, Jamie Eder, Ronni Kass, Rama Kolesnikow, Shelby Campbell, Carlos Ambrozak, Alisa Mast, Timothy Wicks, Patsy Creedy, Jeffrey Schneider, Line Dam, Emilia De Marchis, Aaron Eash, Nettie Pardue, Jeff Pflueger, and Tara Kini. Space does not permit me to mention all the wonderful people who have touched and enriched my life: please know that I appreciate you.

Finally, I would like to thank my mother, father, and brother, for the unforgettable life that the four of us once shared in a little town in England: I wouldn't be here without you. Above all, I wish to thank my brilliant wife, my darling daughter, and my astonishing son, for your love; for your forbearance during the many months in which I was secluded at my writing desk; but most of all, for being your spectacular selves.

RESOURCES

If you are in crisis, the following organizations are available to help:

National Suicide Prevention Lifeline
https://suicidepreventionlifeline.org
1-800-273-8255

Substance Abuse and Mental Health Services Administration (SAMHSA) National Helpline
1-800-662-4357

Childhelp National Child Abuse Hotline
https://www.childhelp.org/hotline
1-800-422-4453

National Runaway Safeline
https://www.1800runaway.org/youth-teens
1-800-786-2929

National Association for Children of Addiction
https://nacoa.org
1-888-554-2627

National Alliance on Mental Illness
https://www.nami.org
1-800-950-6264

NOTES

1. *Corpus Hermeticum XI: The Mind to Hermes*, quoted in F. Yates, *Giordano Bruno and the Hermetic Tradition* (London: Univ. of Chicago Press, 1964).
2. A. Dietrich, "Transient Hypofrontality as a Mechanism for the Psychological Effects of Exercise," *Psychiatry Research* 145, no. 1 (2006): 79–83.
3. D. S. Jordan, *The Philosophy of Despair* (San Francisco: Paul Elder and Morgan Shepard, 1902).
4. D. W. Winnicott, "Fear of Breakdown," *International Review of Psycho-Analysis* 1 (1974): 103–7.
5. G. Bruno, *De Umbris Idearum* [On the Shadows of Ideas], trans. S. Gosnell (CreateSpace, 2013; Rome: Aracne, 1582).
6. P. M. Bromberg, "Multiple Self-States, the Relational Mind, and Dissociation: A Psychoanalytic Perspective," in *Dissociation and the Dissociative Disorders: DSM-V and Beyond*, ed. P. F. Dell and J. A. O'Neil (New York: Routledge/Taylor & Francis, 2009), 637–52.
7. E. Nijenhuis, O. van der Hart, and K. Steele, "Trauma-Related Structural Dissociation of the Personality," *Activitas Nervosa Superior* 52, no. 1 (2010): 1–23.
8. E. Husserl, *On the Phenomenology of the Consciousness of Internal Time (1893–1917)*, trans. J. B. Brough (Dordrecht, Netherlands: Kluwer, 1991).
9. J. P. Hamilton, M. Farmer, P. Fogelman, and I. H. Gotlib, "Depressive Rumination, the Default-Mode Network, and the Dark Matter of Clinical Neuroscience," *Biological Psychiatry* 78, no. 4 (2015): 224–30.
10. S. Freud, "On Beginning the Treatment (Further Recommendations on the Technique of Psycho-Analysis I)," in *The Standard Edition of the Complete Psychological Works of Sigmund Freud, Volume XII (1911–1913): The Case of Schreber, Papers on Technique, and Other Works*, ed. J. Strachey (London: Vintage, Hogarth Press, and the Institute of Psycho-Analysis, 2001): 121–44.
11. S. Freud, "Remembering, Repeating, and Working-Through (Further Recommendations on the Technique of Psycho-Analysis II)," in *The Standard Edition of the Complete Psychological Works of Sigmund Freud,*

Volume XII (1911–1913): The Case of Schreber, Papers on Technique, and Other Works, ed. J. Strachey (London: Vintage, Hogarth Press, and the Institute of Psycho-Analysis, 2001): 150–56.

12. B. Jowett, *The Dialogues of Plato: Volume III* (Oxford: Oxford Univ. Press, 1871).

13. J. A. Rumi, *The Essential Rumi*, trans. C. Barks (New York: HarperCollins Publishers, 1995).

14. S. Jha, B. Dong, and K. Sakata, "Enriched Environment Treatment Reverses Depression-like Behavior and Restores Reduced Hippocampal Neurogenesis and Protein Levels of Brain-Derived Neurotrophic Factor in Mice Lacking Its Expression Through Promoter IV," *Translational Psychiatry* 1, no. 9 (2011): e40.

15. K. Dąbrowski, "The Theory of Positive Disintegration," *International Journal of Psychiatry* 2, no. 2 (1966): 229–44.

16. R. L. Carhart-Harris, R. Leech, P. J. Hellyer, M. Shanahan, A. Feilding, E. Tagliazucchi, D. R. Chialvo, and D. Nutt, "The Entropic Brain: A Theory of Conscious States Informed by Neuroimaging Research with Psychedelic Drugs," *Frontiers in Human Neuroscience* 8, no. 1 (2014): article 20.